Introduction to Bronchoscopy

T0134148

Introduction to Bronchoscopy

Second Edition

Edited by

Armin Ernst
St. Elizabeth's Medical Center, Boston, MA

Felix J. F. Herth
Thoraxklinik, University of Heidelberg, Germany

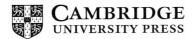

CAMBRIDGE
UNIVERSITY PRESS

University Printing House, Cambridge CB2 8BS, United Kingdom

One Liberty Plaza, 20th Floor, New York, NY 10006, USA

477 Williamstown Road, Port Melbourne, VIC 3207, Australia

4843/24, 2nd Floor, Ansari Road, Daryaganj, Delhi - 110002, India

103 Penang Road, #05-06/07, Visioncrest Commercial, Singapore 238467

Cambridge University Press is part of the University of Cambridge.

It furthers the University's mission by disseminating knowledge in the pursuit of
education, learning and research at the highest international levels of excellence.

www.cambridge.org
Information on this title: www.cambridge.org/9781107449527
DOI: 10.1017/9781316084182

© Cambridge University Press (2009) 2017

First published 2009
Second edition 2017
Reprinted 2022

Printed in the United Kingdom by Print on Demand, World Wide

A catalog record for this publication is available from the British Library

ISBN 978-1-107-44952-7 Paperback

Cambridge University Press has no responsibility for the persistence or accuracy
of URLs for external or third-party internet websites referred to in this publication,
and does not guarantee that any content on such websites is, or will remain,
accurate or appropriate.

. . . .

Every effort has been made in preparing this book to provide accurate and up-to-date
information that is in accord with accepted standards and practice at the time of publication.
Although case histories are drawn from actual cases, every effort has been made to disguise
the identities of the individuals involved. Nevertheless, the authors, editors, and publishers
can make no warranties that the information contained herein is totally free from error, not
least because clinical standards are constantly changing through research and regulation. The
authors, editors, and publishers therefore disclaim all liability for direct or consequential
damages resulting from the use of material contained in this book. Readers are strongly
advised to pay careful attention to information provided by the manufacturer of any drugs or
equipment that they plan to use.

Contents

Contributors

Luis F. Angel, MD
Assistant Professor of Pulmonary Diseases & Critical Care Medicine, the UT Health Science Center at San Antonio

Rabih Bechara, MD, FCCP
Chief of Interventional Pulmonary, Pulmonary, & Critical Care Medicine, Southeastern Regional Medical Center

Heinrich D. Becker, MD
Retired, Thoraxklinik at the University of Heidelberg, Germany

Phillip M. Boiselle, MD
Associate Dean for Academic and Clinical Affairs and Professor of Radiology, Harvard Medical School, Boston

Daniel C. Chelius, Jr., MD
Assistant Professor of Pediatric Otolaryngology – Head and Neck Surgery, Bayor College of Medicine, Houston

Armin Ernst, MD, MHCM
Professor of Medicine, Tufts University School of Medicine, Boston

David Feller-Kopman, MD
Associate Professor of Medicine, John Hopkins, Baltimore

William Fischer, MD
Assistant Professor of Medicine, UNC School of Medicine

Anne L. Fuhlbrigge, MD, MS
Pulmonary and Critical Care Medicine, Brigham and Women's Hospital, Harvard Medical School, Boston

Robert Garland, RRT
Marketing Development Manager/Veran Medical

Jed A. Gorden, MD
Director, Interventional Pulmonology, Swedish Medical Center, Seattle

Dominik Harzheim, MD
Department of Pulmonology and Respiratory Care Medicine, Thoraxklinik at the University of Heidelberg

Felix J. F. Herth, MD, PhD
Professor of Medicine, Department of Pulmonology and Respiratory Care Medicine, Thoraxklinik at the University of Heidelberg

Jonas Herth
Translational Lung Research Center Heidelberg

Shana Hill, MD
The Permanente Medical Group

Rani Kumaran, MD
Northside Pulmonary and Sleep Medicine

Carla Lamb, MD
Director, Interventional Pulmonary, Lahey Clinic MA; Assistant Clinical Professor, Tufts University School of Medicine

Karen S. Lee, MD
Director of Fellowship Training Program, Radiology, Beth Israel Deaconess Medical Center; Assistant Professor of Medicine, Harvard Medical School, Boston

Deborah J. Levine, MD, FCCP
Pulmonary Medicine Clinic, University Transplant Center, University Hospital San Antonio

William Lunn, MD, FACP
President and CEO, Tulane University
Health System, New Orleans

John Pawlowski, MD, PhD
Director, Division of Thoracic Anesthesia,
Beth Israel Deaconess Medical Center,
Boston; Assistant Professor, Harvard
Medical School Boston, MA

Maren Schuhmann, MD, MRCP
Consultant Respiratory Physician,
Department of Pulmonology and Critical
Care Medicine, Thoraxklinik at University
Hospital Heidelberg, Germany

Scott Shofer MD, PhD
Division of Pulmonary, Allergy, and
Critical Care, Duke University Medical
Center Durham, NC

Arthur Wai Sung, MD
Clinical Associate Professor, Medicine,
Stanford University School of Medicine

Melissa Tukey, MD
Assistant Professor of Medicine, Brown
University

Momen M. Wahidi, MD, MBA
Chief Medical Officer, Duke PRMO;
Associate Professor of Medicine, Duke
University

Aaron B. Waxman, MD, PhD
Associate Professor of Medicine, Harvard
Medical School

A Short History of Bronchoscopy

Heinrich D. Becker and Armin Ernst

In his article titled *"Entfernung eines Knochenstücks aus dem rechten Bronchus auf natürlichem Wege und unter Anwendung der directen Laryngoskopie"* in issue No. 38 (September 1897) of *Münchener Medicinische Wochenschrift*, O. Kollofrath, assistant to Gustav Killian at the Poliklinik of Freiburg University, Germany, in the introduction to his report on the first bronchoscopic extraction of a foreign body, wrote, *"On March 30th of this year I had the honor to assist my admired principal, Herrn Prof. Killian in extraction of a piece of bone from the right bronchus. This case is of such peculiarity with respect to its diagnostic and therapeutic importance that a more extensive description seems justified."* To understand this statement, one must consider the state of the art of airway inspection at that time.

The Pre-endoscopic Era

Access to the airways in the living patient was tried already by Hippocrates (460–370 BC), who advised the introduction of a pipe into the larynx of a suffocating patient. Avicenna of Bukhara (about 1000 AD) used a silver pipe for the same purpose. Vesalius' observation around 1542 that the heartbeat and pulsation of the great vessels stopped when he opened the chest of an experimental animal but returned again after he introduced a reed into the airway and inflated the lungs by use of bellows, which mistakenly made him assume that the trachea was part of the circulating system, from which it carried the name τραχυσ ("rough" in Greek language) or *arteria aspera* ("the rough artery" in Latin).

Desault (1744–1795) advised nasotracheal intubation for treatment of suffocation and removal of foreign bodies. For ages, more than half of accidental inhalations of a foreign body caused the death or chronic illness of the patient because of purulent infection, abscess, fistulas, and malnutrition. Diverse instruments have been designed to remove those foreign bodies blindly from the airways via the larynx or a tracheotomy, called "bronchotomy," which was also used for treatment of subglottic stenosis such as caused by diphtheria. Also, until late into the second half of the last century, a tracheotomy also had a high mortality of up to more than 50 percent; methods were developed for blind intubation. When he presented his "Treatise on the Diseases of the Air Passages," Horace Green in 1846, however, was blamed by the Commission of the New York Academy of Medical Sciences as presenting *"... a monstrous assumption, ludicrously absurd, and physically impossible, ... an anatomical impossibility and unwarrantable innovation in practical medicine"* and was removed from the society, but Joseph O'Dwyer persisted and introduced the method for emergency intubation of diphtheric children.

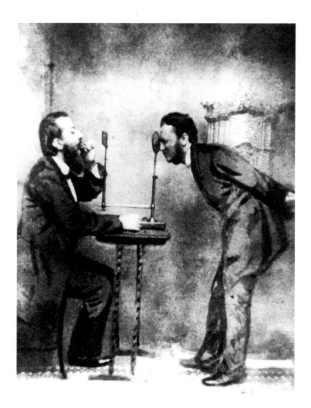

Figure 1.1 Czermak demonstrating the laryngeal mirror.

The Development of Endoscopy

Although instruments for the inspection of the body cavities such as the mouth, nose, ear, vagina, rectum, urethra, and others had been in use for ages, Porter in 1838 still stated, *"There is perhaps no kind of disease covered by greater darkness or posing more difficulties to the practitioner than those of the larynx and the trachea"* because until then the larynx could be only insufficiently inspected by forcible depression of the tongue with a spatula, a so-called "Glossokatochon." Nobody had ever looked into the living trachea. It was only after the advent of three major inventions – (i) instruments for inspection, (ii) suitable light sources, and (iii) sufficient anesthesia – that direct inspection of the airways and visually controlled treatment became possible.

The Laryngeal Mirror

Experiments on the inspection of the larynx with the help of mirrors had been performed, among others, by Latour (1825), Senn (1829), Belloc (1837), Liston (1840), and Avery (1844), but it was not a physician but a singing teacher in London, Manuel Garcia, who in 1854 first observed his own larynx with the help of a dental mirror that he had bought from the French instrument maker Charriére in Paris. Without knowing Garcia's work, laryngologist Ludwig Türck around the same time in 1856 in Vienna performed his first experiment with a similar device, which he borrowed from the physiologist Czermak of Budapest, when in winter the illumination was no longer sufficient for continuation of his studies (Figure 1.1). Czermak reported his findings before Türck, which resulted in a long fight over rights of priority, the so-called "Türkenkrieg" (Turk's war).

With the use of these instruments, diagnosis and treatment of laryngeal diseases became much easier, so that G. D. Gibb in 1862 said, "It has fallen to my lot to see cases of laryngeal disease…that have existed for ten or twenty years, and submitted to every variety of treatment, without the slightest benefit, at the hands of some of the foremost amongst us, wherein the symptoms have depended upon a little growth attached to one or both vocal chords, which was recognized in as many seconds as the complaints had existed years. The nature of the malady thus being made out, the plan of treatment to be pursued became obvious." It was also in 1862 that the German surgeon Victor von Bruns in Tübingen, with the help of this laryngoscopic mirror, could remove the first polyp from a vocal chord in his own brother. Without suitable anesthetics, the procedure needed weeks of preparation by gradual desensitization on the patient's side and much training on anatomical preparations and living larynxes of volunteers. Also his report was rejected as "…a daring deed that should not be imitated and the practical importance of which seems less as there would be hardly another opportunity for its repetition." One of the major problems was the indirect and reverse view of the image, which added to the difficulties.

The First Endoscopes and Light Sources

In contrast to other fields of endoscopy, where daylight or candlelight could be introduced for inspection of the vagina, rectum, urethra, and so on, it was only after Philipp Bozzini, a general practitioner in Frankfurt, had developed his "illuminator" in 1805 that a suitable light source for the inspection of the trachea came within sight. The still somewhat clumsy device consisted of a box containing a candle, the light of which was reflected by a hollow mirror into a "conductor," a split metallic tube that could be spread by a simple mechanism. For the inspection of organs that could not be visualized by direct inspection he used a tube with a mirror for reflection of the light and image.

The first suitable successor was in 1853: the instrument of Desormeaux, who also introduced the word "endoscope" for his instrument to inspect the body cavities (Figure 1.2). It was by Desormeaux's endoscope that A. Kußmaul in 1867–1868 performed the first esophago-scopies. The illumination by spirit, however, was insufficient for the inspection of the stomach. The first suitable gastroscope in 1881 by von Mikulicz and Leiter was a closed optic with lenses and prisms that were electrically illuminated at the distal end by a glowing platinum wire that had to be cooled by a constant flow of water and thus was not suitable for application in the airways.

Esophagoscopy was performed mainly by use of hollow tubes and spatulas that were connected to proximal illumination sources. It was also the Viennese endoscope maker Leiter who in 1886 produced the first so-called panelectroscope, a tube that was connected to a handle that contained an electric bulb and a prism for illumination. The instrument was modified by many specialists, such as Gottstein, who was the first to attach a metal tube in 1891, Rosenheim, who accidentally first passed into the trachea, and Kirstein in Berlin. Kirstein intentionally started to intubate the larynx with the esophagoscope and, after his first experience in 1894, began systematic direct inspection, which he called "autoscopy" (Greek: "αυτοσ," meaning directly without the help of a mirror). "I convinced myself…that one can pass the vocal chords intentionally with a middle sized esophagoscope into the cocainized trachea and right down to the bifurcation; this experience should be eventually fructified."

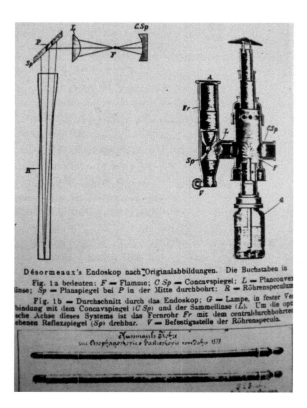

Figure 1.2 An illustration of the Desormeaux endoscope.

But as "the region of the lower trachea is a very dangerous place! ...The rhythmic protrusion of its wall is ...a regular and awe-inspiring phenomenon, which gives cause for utmost care in introducing rigid instruments," he did not "fructify," i.e., expand, his experiments. It was the rhinolaryngologist Gustav Killian of Freiburg University who on June 4, 1895, attended Kirstein's lecture in Heidelberg at the second Congress of the Society of South German Laryngologists, immediately recognized the importance of Kirstein's observation on the diagnosis and treatment of laryngotracheal diseases, and began his experiments with the new method.

In 1877 the urologist Nitze of Dresden and the instrument maker Leiter of Vienna constructed the first lens optic in which electrical illumination was performed by a glowing platinum wire at the distal end that had to be cooled by a constant flow of water when not used inside the urinary bladder, such as in von Mikulicz' first gastroscope. In 1879, T. A. Edison invented the electric bulb, which was further miniaturized by Mignon distal electric illumination to be applied to endoscopy of the airways.

The Development of Local Anesthesia

In his first report on the invention of direct bronchoscopy, Killian said, "Whether one stops inspection with the rigid tube at the bifurcation or passes on for some distance into a major bronchus does not matter for the patient. If he is sufficiently cocainized he does not even realize it." Before the discovery of cocaine, many attempts had been made to anesthetize the airways by use of potassium bromide, ammonia, belladonna, iodine solution, chloroform, morphine, and others. Nothing proved sufficient, and the patients had to be desensitized by weeks of rehearsing touching the pharynx and vocal cords by themselves before a procedure could be performed. The examiner had to be extremely skilled and swift as operations had to be performed within seconds before the view disappeared. Von Bruns suggested training on an excised larynx and on a head that had been severed from a corpse and hung from a hook before training on a volunteer "…who certainly could be found rather easily for a little amount of money and would suffer such not really pleasant but not at all painful or dangerous experiments."

Although Morton in Boston had already introduced general anesthesia by chloroform in 1848, its use was so dangerous that it was only rarely applied in laryngoscopic operations. In 1882, a young scientist at the Pharmacological Institute of Vienna, Sigmund Freud, experimented with cocaine, a sample of which he had bought from Merck Co. He was eager to make a fortune with a breakthrough invention in science to be able to marry his fiancée. But to his later dismay, his experiments in withdrawing morphine addicts from their addiction resulted in disaster. Although he had advised his colleague Koller, an eye specialist, to use a cocaine solution for pain relief when he suffered from severe conjunctivitis, he failed to recognize the importance of his observation himself that cocaine caused numbness when he put it to his tongue. Koller, however, immediately realized the importance of this observation, and after feverishly experimenting with this new "miracle drug" on rabbits and patients, inaugurated local anesthesia in his lecture on September 15, 1884, at the Annual Congress of German Ophthalmologists in Heidelberg. At the same time, the Viennese laryngologist Jellinek introduced cocaine as a local anesthetic for the inspection of the airways: "By eliminating the reflexes of the pharynx and the larynx it was possible to perform some of the operations in which even the most skillful artists in surgery had failed. The procedure completely changed. Virtuosity gave way to careful methodology, skill to exactness, and the former almost endless preparation that so often tried the patience of the physician as well as of the patient could be almost completely abandoned." Thus the way was paved for Gustav Killian to pursue his experiments with bronchoscopy after he had attended Kirstein's lecture in Heidelberg.

Gustav Killian and the Invention of Bronchoscopy

Gustav Killian was born on June 2, 1860, at Mainz on the Rhine. After graduating from high school in 1878, he began to study medicine at the University of Strassburg, where one of his teachers was Adolf Kußmaul. After 1880, he continued clinical education at Freiburg, Berlin, and Heidelberg, where he passed his final examination in 1882. Afterward he started practical work at the municipal hospital of Mannheim close to Heidelberg and later in Berlin to get an education in ENT medicine under the guidance of Hartmann and Fraenkel. As he could not find employment, Killian settled down as a practitioner in Mannheim in 1887. Four months later, he left when he was asked to become head of the section of rhinolaryngology at Freiburg that was part of the large faculty of internal medicine.

At the meeting of the Society of South German Laryngologists in Heidelberg in 1889, he gave a short report on a new technique for examination of the dorsal wall of the larynx. Killian learned about Kirstein's new technique at the meeting of the Laryngological Society in Heidelberg in 1895. Because of the experiences in Krakow of Pieniazek, who had introduced direct lower tracheoscopy via tracheostomy without any complications, Killian at once realized the potential of this new method of direct inspection of the trachea and in 1896 began experimental work. In tracheotomized patients, he passed the bifurcation with the "bronchoscope," a somewhat modified esophagoscope of Rosenheim, and noticed that the bronchi

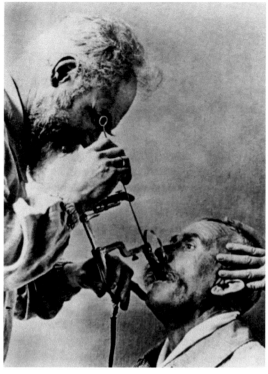

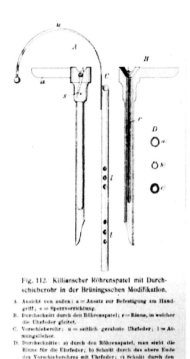

Fig. 112. Killianscher Röhrenspatel mit Durch-
schieberohr in der Brüningsschen Modifikation.

A. Ansicht von außen; a = Ansatz zur Befestigung am Hand-
    griff; s = Sperrvorrichtung.
B. Durchschnitt durch den Röhrenspatel; r = Rinne, in welcher
    die Uhrfeder gleitet.
C. Vorschieberohr; u = seitlich gezahnte Uhrfeder; l = At-
    mungslöcher.
D. Durchschnitte: a) durch den Röhrenspatel, man sieht die
    Rinne für die Uhrfeder; b) Schnitt durch das obere Ende
    des Vorschieberohres mit Uhrfeder; c) Schnitt durch den
    Röhrenspatel nach Einführung des Vorschieberohres.

Figure 1.3 G. Killian performing tracheoscopy with Kasper's electrical handle for illumination attached to his bronchoscope.

were elastic and flexible; he was "stopped only when the diameter of the tube was surpassing that of the bronchi" (Figure 1.3).

After he had confirmed his findings in corpses without tracheotomies as well, he dared to perform the first direct endoscopy via the larynx in a volunteer. He noticed the flexibility of the trachea and how easily he could adjust it to the angle of the main bronchi and introduce the endoscope down to the lobar level. "I think I have made an important discovery," he noted afterwards. Bronchoscopy was born. In the same year (1897), he removed the first foreign body via the translaryngeal route on which his coworker Kollofrath reported in his paper.

After further experience and removal of two more foreign bodies, Killian felt safe to present his new method of "direct bronchoscopy" at the sixth meeting of the Society of South German Laryngologists in Heidelberg on May 29, 1898, and in the same year his first publication on direct bronchoscopy was printed. The following years at Freiburg were full of technical improvements of the new method and the quest for more and more indications of its use. He published 34 papers concerning discovery, technique, and clinical application of his invention. In 1900, he received the award of the Wiener Klinische Wochenschrift for his paper on "Bronchoscopy and its Application in Foreign Bodies of the Lung." Because of his publications and many lectures he was famous, and Freiburg became the Mecca for bronchoscopy. Hundreds of physicians came from all over the world (the list of participants notes 437 foreign guests from all continents, more than 120 from the United States), and up to 20 training courses had to be held every year. He was invited as a popular speaker all over Europe, and patients were sent to him from as far as South America for treatment of foreign bodies, as his son, Hans Killian, a famous surgeon himself, later reported.

To fully understand the importance of endoscopic removal of foreign bodies, one has to consider the state of thoracic surgery in Killian's time. Most patients fell chronically ill after the aspiration of a foreign body, suffering from atelectasis, chronic pneumonia, and hemorrhage (to which half of them succumbed if untreated). Surgical procedures were restricted to pneumotomy when the bronchus was occluded by extensive solid scar tissue and the foreign body could not be reached by the bronchoscope, and it had a very high mortality rate. Lobectomy or pneumonectomy could not be performed before Brunn and Lilienthal developed the surgical techniques for lobectomy after 1910, and Nissen, Cameron Haight, and Graham introduced pneumonectomy after 1930 because techniques in safe closure of the bronchial stump were missing.

Thus for those who were confronted with these patients, it must have seemed like a miracle that already shortly after the introduction of bronchoscopy almost all patients could be cured. According to a statistical analysis of Killian's coworker Albrecht of 703 patients who had foreign bodies aspired during the years 1911–1921, in all but 12 cases the foreign body could be removed bronchoscopically, although many had remained inside the airway for a considerable time; this result showed a success rate of 98.3 percent. In light of this situation, Killian's triumphant remarks become understandable when he states, "One has to be witness when a patient who feels himself doomed to death can be saved by the simple procedure of introducing a tube with the help of a little cocaine. One must have had the experience of seeing a child that at 4 p.m. aspirated a little stone, and that, after the stone has been bronchoscopically removed at 6 p.m., may happily return home at 8 p.m. after anesthesia has faded away. Even if bronchoscopy was ten times more difficult as it really is, we would have to perform it just for having these results."

Besides numerous instruments for foreign body extraction, other devices (e.g., a dilator and even the first endobronchial stent) were constructed. Although the development of bronchoscopy was Killian's main interest in the years at Freiburg, he pushed ahead in other fields, too. He developed the method of submucosal resection of the septum and a new technique for the radical surgery of chronic empyema of the nasal sinuses with resection of the orbital roof and cover by an osseous flap. In about 1906 he began intensive studies of the anatomy and the function of the esophageal orifice, and found the lower part of the m. cricopharyngeus to be the anatomical substrate of the upper esophageal sphincter. According to his observations, it was between this lower horizontal part and the oblique upper part of the muscle (where the muscular layer was thinnest) that Zenker's pulsion diverticulum developed. One of his scholars, Seiffert, later developed a method of endoscopic dissection of the membrane formed by the posterior wall of the diverticulum and the anterior wall of the esophagus.

In 1907 he received an invitation by the American Oto-Rhino-Laryngological Society, and it was on his triumphant journey through the United States that on July 3, 1907, he gave a lecture on these findings at the meeting of the German Medical Society of New York. This lecture was published in *Laryngoscope* in the same year. Lectures were followed by practical demonstrations of his bronchoscopic and surgical techniques and by banquets at night. On his journey he visited Washington, where he had a brief encounter with Theodore Roosevelt. In Pittsburgh he met Chevalier Jackson, then an already outstanding pioneer in esophagobronchology at the University of Pennsylvania. He was awarded the first honorary membership in the Society of American Oto-Rhino-Laryngology and also became an honorary member of the American Medical Association and received a medal in commemoration of his visit.

As Killian was the most famous German laryngologist, when Fraenkel in Berlin retired in 1911 he became successor to the most important chair in rhinolaryngology. Although bronchoscopy seemed to have reached its peak, he felt that visualization of the larynx was unsatisfactory. Using Kirstein's spatula, Killian realized that inspection of the larynx was much easier while the head is in a hanging position, and he had a special laryngoscope constructed that could be fixed to a supporting construction by a hook, a technique he called "suspension-laryngoscopy" by which he could use both hands for manipulation. His coworker Seiffert improved the method by using a chest rest, a technique that later was perfected by Kleinsasser and is still used for endolaryngeal microsurgery.

In 1911, Killian had been nominated Professor at the Kaiser Wilhelm Military Academy of Medicine and, as during World War I, he had to treat laryngeal injuries. He visited the front line in France, where he also met his two sons who were doing service there. After his return from this visit, he founded a center for the treatment of injuries of the larynx and the trachea. During this era he was very much concerned with plastic reconstruction of these organs, especially as he could refer to the work of Dieffenbach and Lexer, two of the most outstanding plastic surgeons of their time, who had also worked in Berlin. The article on the injuries of the larynx would be his last scientific work before he died in 1921 from gastric cancer.

During his last years, Killian prepared several publications on the history of laryngo-tracheobronchoscopy. For teaching purposes, in 1893 he had already begun illustrating his lectures by direct epidiascopic projection of the endoscopic image above the patient's head. Phantoms of the nose, the larynx, and the tracheobronchial tree were constructed according to his suggestions. Because of his always cheerful mood he was called the "semper ridens" (always smiling) and, in his later years, his head being framed by a tuft of white hair, his nickname was "Santa Claus." He founded a school of laryngologists, and his pupils dominated the field of German laryngology and bronchology for years. Albrecht and Brünings published their textbook on direct endoscopy of the airways and esophagus in 1915. Like Carl von Eicken in Erlangen and Berlin and Seiffert in Heidelberg, they had become heads of the most important chairs of oto-rhino-laryngology in Germany. It was to Killian's merit that the separate disciplines of rhinolaryngology and otology were combined. When Killian died on February 24, 1921, his ideas had spread around the world. Everywhere skilled endoscopists developed new techniques, and bronchoscopy became a standard procedure in diagnosis of the airways. His work was the foundation for the new discipline of anesthesiology as well, providing the idea and instruments (laryngoscope by Macintosh) for the access to the airways and endotracheal anesthesia.

Throughout all his professional life, Gustav Killian kept on improving and inventing new instruments and looking for new applications. He applied fluoroscopy, which had been detected by K. Roentgen of Würzburg in 1895, for probing peripheral lesions and foreign bodies. To establish the X-ray anatomy of the segmental bronchi, he introduced bismuth powder. He drained pulmonary abscesses and instilled drugs for clearance via the bronchial route, and he even used the bronchoscope for "pleuroscopy" (thoracoscopy) and transthoracic "pneumoscopy" when abscesses had drained externally. Foreign bodies that had been in place for a long time and had been imbedded by extensive granulations were successfully extracted after treatment of the stenosis by a metallic dilator and, in case of restenosis, metallic or rubber tubes were introduced as stents. Although cancer was a comparatively rare disease (31 primary and 135 secondary cancers in 11,000 postmortems), he pointed out the importance of preoperative and postoperative bronchoscopy. In 1914, he described endoluminal radiotherapy with mesothorium in cancer of the larynx, and in the textbook published in 1915 by his coworkers Albrecht and Brünings, we find the first description of successful curation of a tracheal carcinoma after endoluminal brachyradiotherapy. By taking special interest in teaching his students and assistants to maintain high standards in quality management by constantly analyzing the results of their work and always keeping in mind that he was standing on the shoulders of excellent pioneers, he kept up the tradition of the most excellent scientists in his profession like Billroth, of Vienna. In his inaugural lecture in Berlin on November 2, 1911, he pointed out that it was internal medicine from which the art spread to the other faculties, that patience and empathy should be the main features of a physician, and that one must persist in following one's dreams because "to live means to fight." He ignited the flame of enthusiasm in hundreds of his contemporaries, who spread the technique to other specialties thus founding the roots of contemporary interventional procedures like microsurgery of the larynx (Kleinsasser) and intubation anesthesia (Macintosh, Melzer, and Kuhn).

Rigid Bronchoscopy in the Twentieth Century

Main Schools

Because of the enthusiastic activities of Killian and his assistants in teaching and spreading the new technique, hundreds of specialists all over the world learned bronchoscopy and many improvements were added to the instrument. Thus already by 1910 Killian had collected 1,116 papers – on esophagoscopy (410), gastroscopy (34), and laryngotracheobronchoscopy (672) – for his paper on the history of bronchoscopy and esophagoscopy. It was hardly possible to follow all traits in every continent where, soon after the introduction by pioneers, separate schools developed.

Killian's coworkers von Eicken, Albrecht, Brünings, Seiffert, and others for decades held the chairs of all important departments in Germany. They improved Killian's instruments and introduced new methods such as endoscopic treatment of Zenker's diverticulum by Seiffert, who also developed the chest rest for laryngoscopy (1922), which was perfected by Kleinsasser to the current device for micro-laryngoscopy (1964). Unfortunately after World War II the development took separate ways until recently. In Western Germany, Huzly of Stuttgart was the most prominent researcher in rigid bronchoscopy. In 1961, he edited his photographic atlas of bronchoscopy. Riecker introduced relaxation by curare in 1952, which was replaced with succinylcholine by Mündnich and Hoflehner in 1953. Maassen introduced bronchography via double-lumen catheter in 1956. Two companies, Storz and Wolf, became the most important instrument makers in Germany and introduced new technologies such as the Hopkins telescope and television cameras. E. Schiepatti of Buenos Aires wrote about transtracheal puncture of the carinal lymph nodes, and Euler reported on pulmonary and aortic angiography by transbronchial puncture in 1948–1949 and later on the technique of rigid transbronchial needle aspiration (TBNA) for mediastinal masses in 1955, which was further perfected by Schießle in 1962.

In the United States, where A. Coolidge (on May 11, 1898) performed the first lower tracheobronchoscopy at Massachusetts General Hospital, it was Chevalier Jackson in

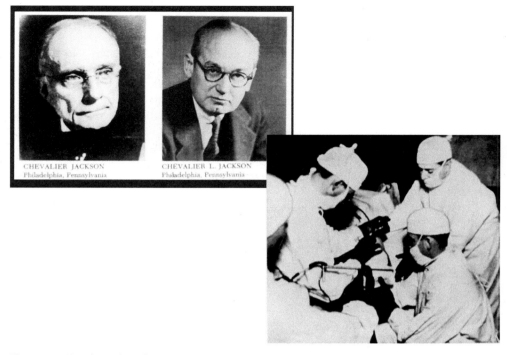

Figure 1.4 Chevalier Jackson, father and son, and introduction of the bronchoscope with laryngoscope.

Philadelphia (whom Killian had met on his visit to the United States in 1907) who, with his instrument maker Pillings, made many improvements in instruments for bronchoscopy and esophagoscopy and became the "father of American bronchoesophagology" (Figure 1.4). During his training to become a laryngologist he had visited London in 1886 where he was shown the "impractical device designed by Morel Mackenzie in an effort visually to inspect the esophagus." In 1890 he constructed the first endoscope "worthy of the name" for esophagoscopy and in 1904 he constructed the first American bronchoscope. After Einhorn in New York had added an integrated light conductor and Fletcher Ingals of Chicago had introduced distal illumination to the esophagoscope, Jackson equipped his bronchoscope with a light carrier with a miniaturized electric Mignon bulb at the distal end and an additional suction channel. Confronted by many patients suffering from aspiration of foreign bodies, he invented many instruments for retrieval. In 1907 he published the first systematic textbook on bronchoesophagology, which he dedicated to Gustav Killian, the "father of bronchoscopy." In this book he addressed modern issues of quality management such as analysis and prevention of complications, rational construction of bronchoscopy suites, and arrangement of equipment and staff. Being a philanthropist, he constantly refused to have his inventions patented as he wanted them to be spread as widely as possible, and by his persistence with the government he pushed for a law for the prevention of accidents by ingestion of caustic agents. He was a perfectionist in techniques and was totally convinced that teaching had to be performed on animals before patients were treated. Therefore, he always refused to go back to England where animal rights activists prevented such training courses. In 1928, in recognition of his "conspicuous achievements in the broad field of

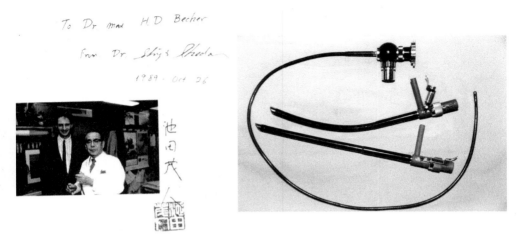

Figure 1.5 S. Ikeda demonstrating the first prototype of the flexible bronchofiberscope to the author. In the transition from rigid to flexible technology he introduced the fiber-scope via an orotracheal tube that could be fixed in a straight position for introduction of a rigid optic and forceps if flexible biopsy was insufficient.

surgical science," the Boston Surgical Society awarded him the Bigelow Medal, which was presented to him by H. Cushing "for his eminent performances and creative power by which he opened new fields of endeavor" and in acknowledgment of his "indefinable greatness of personality." He simultaneously held five chairs of laryngology at different hospitals in his hometown (Pittsburgh) and in Philadelphia. His son Ch. L. Jackson also became a laryngologist and was his successor at Temple University in Philadelphia. He was the founder of the Pan American Association of Otorhinolaryngology and Bronchology and of the International Bronchoesophagological Society, and was cofounder of the World Medical Association. With his father he edited the last issue of the textbook.

Their school extends well into our time as many of today's specialists' teachers were trained by the Jacksons, such as E. Broyles in Baltimore, who after additional training by Haslinger in Vienna introduced the telescope optic for bronchoscopy in 1940, the optical forceps in 1948, and fiber illumination for the rigid bronchoscope in 1962. His student G. Tucker became professor at Jefferson in Philadelphia, where he trained B. Marsh who keeps the tradition alive today along with Ch. M. Norris. P. Hollinger and Brubaker, who became specialists in pediatric bronchoscopy, introduced color photography in the 1940s. Hollinger's son is now a famous pediatric laryngologist. Andersen was the first to perform bronchoscopic transbronchial lung biopsy (TBLB) via the rigid bronchoscope in 1965. Sanders in 1967 introduced jet ventilation for rigid bronchoscopy.

After staying with Killian in Freiburg, it was Inokichi Kubo of Kyushu University in Fukuoka who first introduced bronchoscopy to Japan in 1907. He was joined by S. Chiba who, after training with Brünings, stayed in Tokyo from 1910. Joe Ono (who was trained by Jackson in 1934) founded the Japan Broncho-Esophagological Society in 1949. Shigeto Ikeda, who later developed the flexible fiberscope, introduced glasfiber illumination for the rigid bronchoscope in 1962 (Figure 1.5). When Ikeda, who found rigid bronchoscopy under local anesthesia in the sitting position on "Killian's chair" cumbersome, introduced the flexible bronchoscope, he used it in combination with a flexible tube that could be straightened by

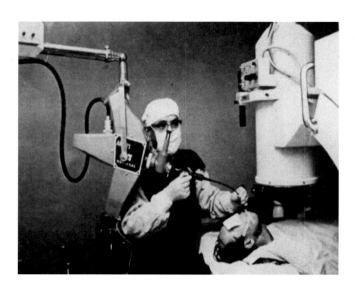

Figure 1.6 S. Ikeda with film camera attached to the fiberscope.

a locking mechanism so that he was still able to introduce the rigid optic in the same session. In the era of expanding interventional procedures, this method of combining both the rigid and the flexible endoscope today regains new attention (Figure 1.6).

Technical Developments

ILLUMINATION. After the advent of the electric bulb, illumination became sufficient for the illumination of the airways. At first the lamps were installed separately on statives or fixed to a headrest from where the light was reflected into the endoscope. Connection of the light source to the endoscope improved handling considerably. Thus Killian and his coworkers preferred to use Casper's panelectroscope, in which the light bulb was integrated into the handle from where it was reflected by a prism to the endoscope, because it was not so easily soiled by secretions. Jackson, however, used distal illumination via a light guide with a Mignon bulb at its tip. By the late 1880s, von Schrötter in Vienna had developed a rigid light guide made of Plexiglas, which was improved by K. Storz, who introduced quartz. After Tyndall's first description of the optical properties of glass fibers in 1872, patents for glass fibers as a transport medium were almost simultaneously given to Baird in England (1926), Hansell in the United States (1927), and Marconi in England (1930). The first prototype of a fiberscope was presented by Lamm in Munich (1930). After Hansen in Denmark described the first fiber bundles for light transportation in 1930, van Heel in the Netherlands and O'Brian in the United States developed the first endoscopes for bronchoscopy and gastroscopy in 1953 and 1954. The rod lens and fiber-optic lighting device by Hopkins in London was adopted by K. Storz as a cold light illumination source for his rigid endoscopes in 1963. The transition to fully flexible endoscopes with image transport by glass fibers was performed by Hirschowitz and American Cystoscope Makers, Inc (ACMI) in 1958 after Curtiss of Ann Arbor had described the first medical fiber instrument in 1955.

PHOTO-, FILM-, AND VIDEODOCUMENTATION. The first (even stereoscopic) endophotographies were performed by Czermak by use of a giant laryngeal mirror (Figure 1.1). Stein in Frankfurt used magnesia illumination for his photographic apparatus, the "heliopictor" (ca. 1875), technically the predecessor of the Polaroid Land Camera of 100 years later. Stein's camera was improved by Nitze and Kollmann. In 1907, Benda introduced color photography, which was first introduced by P. Hollinger to bronchoscopy in 1941. Soulas (1949) and Hollinger (1956) also introduced endoscopic film documentation. The first television transmission of a bronchoscopy was performed by Dubois de Monternaud in 1955. Wittmoser constructed an angulated optic for improving image transfer and produced the first video documentation in 1969.

Prospects

With the advent of the flexible bronchoscope after 1966, two developments took place: Bronchoscopy rapidly spread beyond otorhinolaryngological and specialized thoracic clinics, and the overall number of rigid bronchoscopies declined rapidly until the late 1980s and early 1990s because bronchoscopy had become much easier. Then again, the increasing number of interventional techniques demanded use of the rigid bronchoscope for safety reasons. Special rigid devices were developed by J. F. Dumon for application of the Nd:YAG (neodymium-doped yttrium aluminum garnet) laser and placement of his "dedicated stent" and by L. Freitag for his "dynamic stent." Consensus task forces of the Scientific Section of Endoscopy of the German Society for Pulmonology and of the European Respiratory Society/American Thoracic Society (ERS/ATS), as well as the American College of Chest Physicians (ACCP), agreed that for many interventional procedures the bronchoscopist and staff should at least be trained in the technique of rigid bronchoscopy and should have the instrument at hand in case of an emergency. Thus in training courses all over the world, handling of the rigid instrument is taught again.

Flexible Bronchoscopy

Broad application of bronchoscopy took place only following the development of flexible instruments that could be easily introduced under local anesthesia. The pioneer of this technique was Shigeto Ikeda at the National Cancer Center Hospital in Tokyo, Japan. After Kubo and Ono had introduced rigid bronchoscopy and the related technologies to Japan, Ikeda became the proponent of bronchoscopy and pioneer in flexible bronchoscopy. Fiber technology had been introduced to gastrointestinal endoscopy quite some time before. Glasfiber bundles were used for illumination by cold light to replace bulbs at the tip of endoscopes, which produced considerable heat and potential damage. In addition, instruments themselves became flexible and made inspection of the organs easier. The first application was in connection with gastrocameras that had a small photographic lens system at their tip with miniature films that could be analyzed by viewing with a projector. With the reduction in fiber size and improvement of fiber arrangement, imaging via optic fiber bundles became possible, allowing real time inspection and instrumentation under visual control. However, the diameter of these instruments was too big for introduction into the airways.

Shigeto Ikeda and the Development of the Fiberscope

Shigeto Ikeda, born in 1925, decided to become a specialist in thoracic medicine after recovering from tuberculosis at the age of 23 and started his education in thoracic surgery. In 1962 he joined the National Cancer Center in Tokyo where he also performed rigid bronchoscopy for diagnosis of lung cancer, using among other instruments the curette, developed by Tsuboi. For better illumination in esophagoscopy, he had fiber glass light transmission applied to the rigid optics. With regard to the flexibility of the fibers and the experiences that had been made with fiber optics in gastroenterology, he considered having the technique also applied in bronchoscopes. Thus in 1962 he approached Mr. Machida and asked for the development of a flexible bronchofiberscope with a diameter of less than 6 mm, containing approximately 15,000 glass fibers of less than 15 μm. In 1964 he obtained the first prototype of this device and, after further improvement in the summer of 1966, he was able to present the first useful instrument at a meeting in Copenhagen. The new device was reported as a sensation in the *New York Times*. After further technical improvements to enhance maneuvering and image quality (and including a biopsy channel for taking biopsies) the Machida flexible broncho-scope became commercially available in 1968, which can be considered the year of the second revolution in bronchoscopy, as bronchoscopy spread beyond specialized centers worldwide. Shortly afterward in 1970 the first Olympus model was commercialized with better handling and imaging properties. In 1968 Ikeda demonstrated the new instrument at many interna-tional meetings and presented it to the National Institutes of Health (NIH) and to the Mayo Clinic in Rochester, Minnesota, where he learned about the Mayo mass screening project for early detection of lung cancer in 1970. This was the inspiration for establishing several screening projects in Japan.

Eager to spread the technique of flexible bronchoscopy with the fiberscope, Ikeda orga-nized several additional groups for investigation and many training courses. In 1975 the Anti-Lung Cancer Association was founded in Japan for early detection in smokers over 40 years old. To enhance the understanding and systematic approach with the fiber bronchoscope, Ikeda developed new terminology for the bronchial tree and delicate models for training, especially in X-ray interpretation. The flexible bronchoscope was applied worldwide, and the vast majority of bronchoscopies were performed by this technique under local anesthesia. In 1978 Ikeda organized the first World Congress for Bronchology (WCB) in Tokyo, and in 1979 he founded the World Association for Bronchology (WAB), of which he was elected the first chairman. In 1983 the Japan Society for Bronchology (JSB) was inaugurated.

Ikeda never stopped improving the instrument and developing new techniques in con-nection with flexible bronchoscopy. His next major achievement was the introduction of a video technique, which he began investigating in 1983 and finally could commercialize in 1987. In 1989 Ikeda suffered a cerebral ischemic insult and more followed, as well as several heart infarctions, to which he finally succumbed on December 25, 2001.

In Japan several enthusiastic doctors applied flexible bronchoscopy for introduction of new techniques. Among those pioneers were Arai, performing transbronchial lung biopsies; Kato, treating early lung cancer by photodynamic therapy (PDT); and Watanabe, introducing the spigot for treatment of bronchial fistulas. With the increase of interventional procedures, the necessity for reintroduction of rigid bronchoscopy to combine with the flexible broncho-scope became obvious, and in 1998 Miyazawa organized the first international conference for this purpose in Hiroshima (Figure 1.7).

Further Developments in Flexible Bronchoscopy

The ease of application and of access beyond the central airways opened vast opportunities for introduction of new optical, diagnostic, and therapeutic techniques, starting with TBLB, performed by Anderson and Zavala after Ikeda's visit to the United States. In 1974, H. Reynolds published his first experiences with bronchoalveolar lavage (BAL). D. Cortese demonstrated the potential of early lung cancer detection by fluorescence, induced by injection of hematoporphyrin derivatives (HPDs) in 1978. In the same year, K. P. Wang

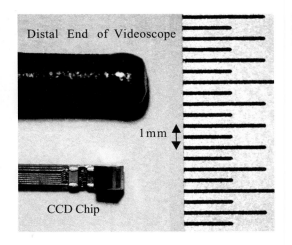

Distal End of Videoscope

1 mm

CCD Chip

Figure 1.7 Tips of a regular adult video bronchoscope in comparison with an ultrathin bronchoscope.

had started performing TBNA of mediastinal lymph nodes via the flexible bronchoscope, which by then was only rarely applied via rigid instruments. Also, the first endobronchial application of the Nd:YAG laser was performed by Toty in the same year, and in 1980 J. F. Dumon published his results in photoablation of stenoses by Nd:YAG laser treatment, which afterward became the most applied technique for a long time. In parallel Y. Hayata and H. Kato applied PDT after sensitization by HPD for treatment of centrally located early lung cancer. In 1979 Hilarss used radioactive probes for treatment of central airway cancer for endoscopic high-dose radiation therapy. With rapid development and miniaturization of electronic imaging by charge-coupled device chips, the first video bronchoscope was developed by Ikeda in cooperation with Pentax in 1987 (Figure 1.8). Two years later, in 1990, the first dedicated stent for the airways was presented by J. F. Dumon, and in 1991 S. Lam reported on autofluorescence bronchoscopy without HPD for early detection of lung cancer. The need for local staging of these lesions was met by the introduction of endobronchial ultrasound (EBUS) in 1999 (Becker), which in addition opened a wide range of applications for diagnosis within the mediastinum and the lung and currently, in connection with TBNA by a dedicated ultrasonic bronchoscope (2003), is beginning to replace mediastinoscopy for staging of lung cancer. Early detection of lung cancer created further demand for new imaging modalities by high-power magnification videobronchoscopes and narrow band imaging for analysis of subtle vascular structures (Shibuya 2002). Endoscopic optical coherence tomography providing information of the layer structure of the bronchial wall with higher resolution than EBUS (Fujimoto 2002) is currently under investigation for bronchology. Maneuvering smart diagnostic tools inside the airways beyond the visible range has been enhanced by smart electromagnetic navigation (2003), which also supported bronchoscopic treatment of peripheral lesions by insertion of brachytherapy catheters (2005). Recently, endobronchial treatment of asthma by thermal destruction of the bronchial muscles, has been approved for use and different forms of endobronchial lung volume rediction continue to be explored and used (2007). The rapid growth of internet opened new ways for communication to enhance consulting, research, and teaching.

The exponential increase in computer capacity will create a wide range of new techniques that will also affect bronchology in the near future with regard to diagnostic and therapeutic

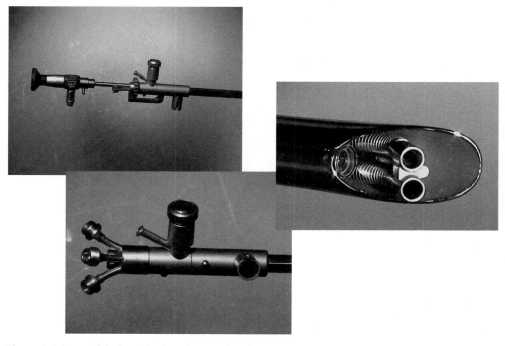

Figure 1.8 Image of the first video bronchoscope (1987).

procedures, and within the next decade bronchoscopy will gain even more importance in pulmonary medicine than it already has by now, 110 years after its invention.

Further Readings

Becker HD. Gustav Killian – a biographical sketch. *J Bronchol*. 1995;2:77–83.

Becker HD. The impact of current technological development on bronchoscopy. *J Japan Bronchoesophagological Soc*. 2004;55(2):89–91.

Becker HD. Bronchoscopy and computer technology. In: Simoff MJ, Sterman DH, Ernst A, eds. *Thoracic Endoscopy: Advances in Interventional Pulmonology*. Malden, MA: Blackwell Publishers; 2006:88–118

Kollofrath O. Entfernung eines Knochenstücks aus dem rechten Bronchus auf natürlichem Wege und unter Anwendung der directen *Laryngoskopie*. *MMW Munch Med Wochenschr*. 1897;38:1038–1039.

Becker HD, Marsh BR. History of the rigid bronchoscope. In: Bolliger CT, Mathur PN, eds. *Interventional Bronchoscopy, Prog Respir Res*. Basel: Karger; 2000:2–15, 30.

Brandt HJ. *Endoskopie der Luft- und Speisewege*. Berlin: Springer; 1985.

Brünings W, Albrecht W. *Direkte Endoskope der Luft- und Speisewege. Neue Deutsche Chirurgie Bd.16*. Stuttgart: F. Enke; 1915.

Byck R. *Cocaine Papers by Sigmund Freud*. New York: Stonehill; 1974.

Cushing H. Boston Surgical Society: The presentation of the Henry Jacob Bigelow Medal. *N Engl J Med*. 1928;199:16.

Czermak J. *Physologische Untersuchungen mit Garcia's Kehlkopfspiegel.* Vienna: K. Gerold's Sohn; 1858.

Elsberg L. *Laryngoscopal Medication or the Local Treatment of the Diseases of the Throat, Larynx, and Neighboring Organs, under Sight.* New York: William Wood & Co.; 1864.

Garcia M. *Beobachtungen über die Menschliche Stimme.* Vienna: W. Braunmüller; 1878.

Gibb GD. *The Laryngoscope: Illustrations of its Practical Application, and Description of its Mechanism.* London: J. Churchill & Sons; 1863.

Hayata Y, Kato H, Konaka C, Ono J, Takizawa N. Haematoporphyrine derivate and laser photoradiation in the treatment of lung cancer. *Chest.* 1982;81:269–277.

Huzly A. *Atlas der Bronchoskopie.* Stuttgart: G. Thieme; 1960.

Ikeda S. The development and progress of endoscopes in the field of bronchoesophagology. *JJSB.* 1988;39:85–96.

Ikeda S, Yanai N. Flexible bronchofiberscope. *Kejo J Med.* 1968;17:1–16.

Jackson C. *The Life of Chevalier Jackson. An Autobiography.* New York: Macmillan; 1938.

Jackson C, Jackson CL. *Bronchoesophagology.* Philadelphia and London: W.B. Saunders Co.; 1950.

Killian G. Ueber directe bronchoscopie. *MMW Munch Med Wochenschr.* 1898;27:844–847.

Killian G. Description abrégée de mon operation radicale sur le sinus frontal. *Asnn Mal Oreille Larynx.* 1902;28:205–209.

Killian G. *Bronchoskopie und Lungenchirurgie. Verh Verein Südd Laryngologen.* Wurzburg: Stuber's Verlag; 1905.

Killian G. Tracheo-bronchoscopy in its diagnostic and therapeutical aspects. *Laryngoscope.* 1906;12: 3–15.

Killian G. Über die Behandlung von Fremdkörpern unter Bronchialstenosen. *Zschr Ohrenheilk.* 1907; 15:334–370.

Killian G. Über den Mund der Speiseröhre. *Zschr Ohrenkheilk.* 1907;55:1–41.

Killian G. Zur Geschichte der Bronchoskopie und Ösophagoskopie. *DMW.* 1911;35:1585–1687.

Killian G. Die directen Methoden in den Jahren 1911 und 1912. *Semon's Internat Centralbl Laryngol Rhinol.* 1913;30:1–28.

Killian G. Zwei Falle von Karzinom. *Berlin Klin Wochenschr.* 1914;7:1–3.

Killian G. Zur Geschichte der Endoskopie von den ältesten Zeiten bis Bozzini. *Arch Laryngol.* 1915;29: 247–393.

Killian G. *Die Schwebelaryngoskopie und ihre Klinische Verwertung.* Berlin: Urban und Schwarzenberg; 1920.

Killian H. A model for bronchoscopy. Translation of a paper in *Archiv für Laryngologie* 13:1, Berlin 1902. Harvard, derby, 1902.

Killian H. *Hinter uns Steht nur der Herrgott. Aufzeichnungen eines Chirurgen. Sub Umbra Dei.* Munich: Kindler; 1957.

Killian H. *Gustav Killian. Sein Leben. Sein Werk.* Remscheid-Lennep: Dustri Verlag; 1958.

Kirstein A. Autoskopie des Larynx und der Trachea (besichtigung ohne spegel). *Berlin KliWschr.* 1895; 22:476–478.

Kluge F. Die Erstanwendung der Ösophago- und Gastroskopie durch A. Kußmaul und seine Assistenten 1868. *Fortschr Gastroenterol Endoskope.* 1986;15:5–9.

Marsh BR. Historic development of bronchoesophagology. *Otolaryngol Head Neck Surg.* 1996;114: 689–716.

Mikulicz J. *Über Gastroskopie und Ösophagoskopie.* Vienna: Urban & Schwarzenberg; 1881.

Miyazawa T. History of the flexible bronchoscope. In: Bolliger CT, Mathur PN, eds. *Interventional Bronchoscopy. Prog Respir Res.* Basel: Karger; 2000;30:16–21.

Naef HP. *The Story of Thoracic Surgery.* Toronto: Hogrefe and Huber; 1990.

Ohata M. History and progress of bronchology in Japan. *JJSB.* 1998;20:539–546.

Pieniazek P. Die tracheoskopie und die tracheoskopischen operationen bei tracheotomierten. *Arch Laryngol.* 1896;28:210–230.

Reuter HJ, Reuter MA. *Philipp Bozzini und die Endoskopie des 19.Jh.* Stuttgart: Loennicker; 1988.

Richard P. *Notice sur l'Invention du Laryngoscope ou mroirs du Larynx (Garcia's Kehlkopfspiegel du Dr. Czermak).* Paris: J. Claye; 1861.

Shirakawa T. The History of Bronchoscopy in Japan. Key Note Lecture, The 12th WCB&WCBE, June 18, 2002, Boston, MA. CD edited by the WAB.

Trousseau A, Belloc H. *Traité Pratique de la Phtisie Laryngeé.* Paris: J.B. Baillière; 1837.

Tsuboi E, Ikeda S. Transbronchial biopsy smear for diagnosis of peripheral pulmonary carcinomas. *Cancer.* 1967;20:687–698.

Türck L. *Klinik der Krankheiten des Kehlkopfes und der Luftröhre nebst einer Anleitung zum Gebrauch des Kehlkopfrachenspiegels und zur Localbehandlung der Kehlkopfkrankheiten.* Vienna: W. Braunmüller; 1866.

Von Bruns V. *Die Laryngoskopie und die Laryngoskopische Chirurgie.* Tübingen: H. Laupp'sche Buchhandlung; 1865.

von Eicken C. *Zur Geschichte der Endoskopie der oberen Luft- und Speisewege.* Giessen: v. Münchow'sche Universitätsdruckerei; 1921.

Wiesner B. De entwicklung der bronchoskope und der bronchologie. Ein geschichtlicher überblick. *Atemw.- Lungenkrankh.* 1995;21(11)541–547.

2

Multidetector Computed Tomography Imaging of the Central Airways

Karen S. Lee and Phillip M. Boiselle

Introduction

Multidetector computed tomography (MDCT) has emerged as the primary imaging modality for the assessment of the central airways. Current generation MDCT scanners can provide high-spatial-resolution images of the entire central airways in just a matter of seconds, and exceptional quality two-dimensional (2D) multiplanar and three-dimensional (3D) reformation images can be generated simply in a few minutes. MDCT imaging is particularly useful for the evaluation of airway stenoses, endobronchial neoplasms, and complex congenital airway disorders. In addition to providing exquisite anatomic detail of the tracheobronchial tree, the use of dynamic expiratory MDCT imaging can provide important functional information about the airways, including the diagnosis of tracheobronchomalacia. Furthermore, MDCT has become a pivotal imaging tool for the bronchoscopist both pre-procedurally, by helping to plan and guide bronchoscopic procedures, and postprocedurally, by providing a noninvasive imaging method for follow-up after interventions.

Multidetector Computed Tomography Imaging: Axial, 2D Multiplanar, and 3D Reconstruction Images

MDCT-acquired, high-spatial-resolution axial images provide exquisitely detailed anatomic and pathologic information about the airways. The precise size and shape of the airway lumen (Figure 2.1), as well as the presence and distribution of airway wall thickening and/or calcification, can be clearly illustrated (Figure 2.2). Conventional axial images also help to define the relationship of the airways to adjacent structures and extraluminal abnormalities not visible on bronchoscopy.

Evaluation of the airways solely with axial MDCT images, however, can be limiting and challenging. On axial MDCT images, subtle airway stenoses can escape detection, craniocaudal extent of airway disease may be underestimated, and complex airway anatomy may not be clearly defined.

Two-dimensional multiplanar reformations and 3D reconstructions can overcome the limitations of axial MDCT imaging by displaying the airways in a more anatomically meaningful representation. Multiplanar reformation images are single-voxel-thick sections that can be displayed in the coronal, sagittal, or oblique plane. Curved reformations along the axis of the airway can also be obtained, thereby allowing for multiple contiguous airway segments to be simultaneously and completely imaged on a single section. Multiple adjacent thin slices can be added together to form a thick slab image or multiplanar volume reformation image, which typically varies from 5 mm to 10 mm in thickness. These multiplanar

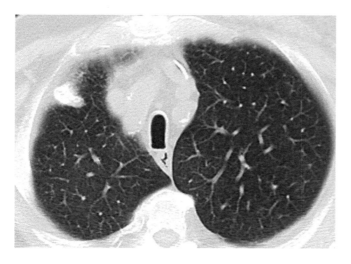

Figure 2.1 Saber-sheath trachea. Axial, noncontrast MDCT image through the intrathoracic trachea demonstrates narrowing of the airway in the transverse dimension with inward bowing of the lateral walls and widening of the airway in the anteroposterior dimension. Saber-sheath trachea is commonly associated with chronic obstructive pulmonary disease.

volume reformation images advantageously combine the high spatial resolution imaging of multiplanar reformation images with the anatomic display of thick slabs (Figure 2.3). Additionally, the use of minimal intensity projection can improve visualization of the airways within the lung parenchyma by emphasizing low-attenuation voxels. These 2D MDCT image reformation techniques allow for easier identification of airway stenosis, precise delineation of the extent of airway disease in multiple planes, and clarification of complex congenital airway abnormalities. Furthermore, because these images are more visually accessible than conventional axial MDCT images, communication among the radiologist, pulmonologist, and patient can be facilitated.

Three-dimensional reconstructed images, including external and internal rendering of the airways, play an important complementary role to conventional bronchoscopy by providing detailed bronchographic and bronchoscopic road map images of the airways. External 3D

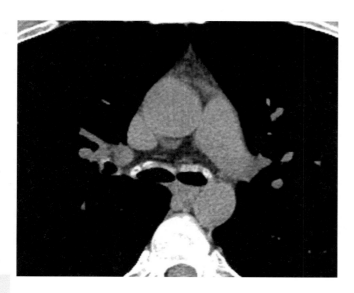

Figure 2.2 Relapsing polychondritis. Axial, noncontrast MDCT image through the main stem bronchi demonstrates smooth calcification and thickening of the anterolateral aspects of the airway wall with characteristic sparing of the posterior membranous wall.

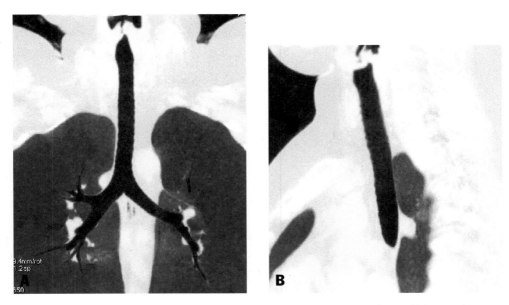

Figure 2.3 Normal 2D multiplanar volume reformations of the airways. Coronal **(A)** and sagittal **(B)** minimal intensity projection images demonstrating normal appearance of the central airways.

rendering of the airways, or CT bronchography, displays the external surface of the airways and its relationship to adjacent structures (Figure 2.4). These images improve conspicuity of subtle airway stenoses and enhance the display and characterization of complex congenital airway abnormalities. Internal 3D rendering of the airways, or virtual bronchoscopy, allows the viewer to navigate through the internal lumen of the airways, providing a prospective

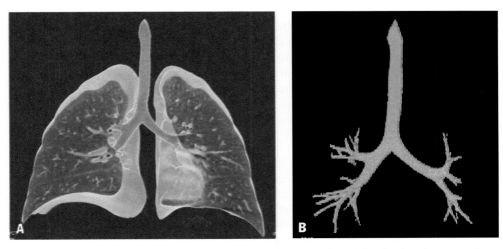

Figure 2.4 Normal 3D external renderings of the airways with lung parenchyma **(A)** and without lung parenchyma **(B)**. Exclusion of lung parenchyma highlights segmental bronchial anatomy.

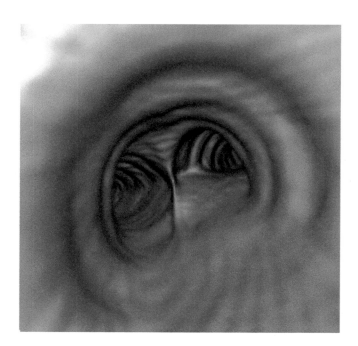

Figure 2.5 Normal 3D internal rendering of the airways. Virtual bronchoscopy image simulates conventional bronchoscopic view of the distal trachea and carina.

similar to conventional bronchoscopy (Figure 2.5). These virtual bronchoscopic images can provide important complementary information to bronchoscopy by assessing the airways distal to a high-grade stenosis, beyond which a conventional bronchoscope cannot pass, and by providing a unique, global, 360-degree assessment of endoluminal lesions.

Multidetector Computed Tomography Imaging of Central Airway Pathology

MDCT has become the initial diagnostic modality in the evaluation of many patients suspected of having a central airway abnormality. MDCT can quickly and noninvasively determine if the tracheobronchial tree is anatomically normal, or if an extraluminal, intraluminal, or even functional abnormality of the airway is present. In the following sections, the role of MDCT with 2D and 3D reformation imaging in the evaluation of airway stenoses, central airway neoplasms, and congenital airway abnormalities will be discussed, as well as the use of dynamic expiratory MDCT in the diagnosis of tracheobronchomalacia.

Airway Stenoses

MDCT-generated 2D multiplanar reformation images of the airways are crucial for accurate imaging evaluation of airway stenoses. Multiplanar volume reformation images, in particular, can highlight the presence of mild stenoses, precisely delineate the length of the airway stenoses, and identify the presence of intraluminal horizontal webs (Figure 2.6). These 2D reformation techniques not only provide important information for preprocedural planning prior to airway stent placement or surgery, but also allow for an accurate, noninvasive method of follow-up for these patients postprocedure.

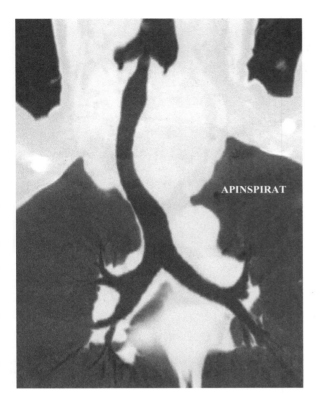

Figure 2.6 Extrinsic airway compression from goiter. Coronal 2D reformation image displays the severity and craniocaudal extent of airway narrowing involving the intrathoracic and extrathoracic trachea due to a large goiter.

In addition to 2D image reformations, both external and internal 3D renderings of the airways have been shown to be important postprocessing techniques for the complete imaging assessment of airway stenosis. As shown in a study by Remy-Jardin and colleagues, external 3D reconstructions, when compared with axial CT imaging alone, can provide important additional information about airway stenoses and allow for more accurate depiction of the length, shape, and severity of airway narrowing (Figure 2.7). In recent years, virtual bronchoscopy has become a rapidly emerging technique for the evaluation of airway stenosis, as this method provides an intraluminal perspective of the airways distal to an area of high-grade luminal narrowing, beyond where a flexible bronchoscope can pass. Furthermore, virtual bronchoscopy can depict airway stenoses from a distal viewpoint, thereby allowing for a comprehensive depiction of the airway narrowing from multiple perspectives (Figure 2.8).

MDCT imaging with 2D multiplanar and 3D reconstruction techniques has been shown to be a highly sensitive, specific, and accurate method for the detection and diagnosis of airway stenoses when compared with flexible bronchoscopy, with reported sensitivities ranging from 87 percent to 92 percent and specificities ranging from 86 percent to 95 percent. In addition, Hoppe and colleagues demonstrated that 2D sagittal reformatted images and virtual bronchoscopic images were more accurate than axial MDCT images alone in the detection of bronchoscopically confirmed central airway stenoses, with accuracies of 96.5, 98, and 96 percent, respectively. These findings underscore the added value of 2D multiplanar and 3D reconstructions in the MDCT imaging evaluation of airway narrowing.

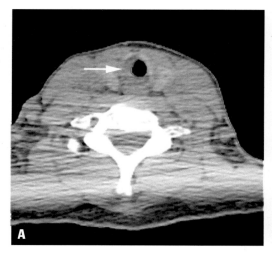
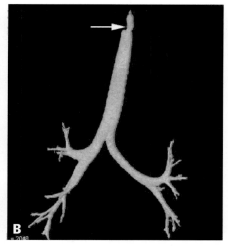

Figure 2.7 Airway stenosis caused by inflammatory bowel disease. **(A)** Axial, non-contrast MDCT image of the sub-glottic trachea demonstrates subtle narrowing of the airway (*arrow*) due to smooth soft tissue thickening along the right lateral and posterior aspects of the tracheal wall. **(B)** External 3D rendering of the central airways more clearly depicts the location and severity of subglottic tracheal stenosis (*arrow*).

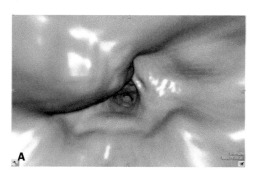
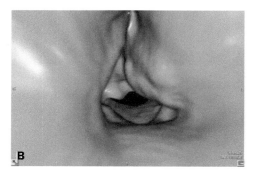

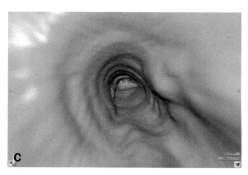

Figure 2.8 Amyloidosis. Virtual bronchoscopic images demonstrate high-grade, irregular narrowing of the proximal trachea due to amyloidosis from both proximal **(A)** and distal **(B)** perspectives. **(C)** Virtual bronchoscopic image obtained at a level distal to the stenosis shows diffuse airway abnormality with patency of the distal trachea and carina.

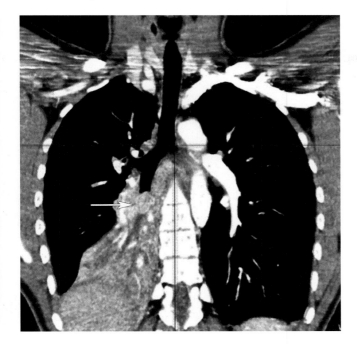

Figure 2.9 Endobronchial carcinoid tumor. Coronal multiplanar reformatted image shows a predominantly intraluminal, enhancing, round mass (*arrow*) obstructing the right lower lobe bronchus resulting in lobar collapse.

Central Airway Neoplasms

MDCT is the imaging modality of choice for the diagnosis, staging, and preoperative planning of central airway neoplasms. The sensitivity of MDCT for identifying airway abnormalities, including neoplasms, is 97 percent. MDCT allows for accurate determination of the 3D size, including craniocaudal length, and precise location of the tumor within the airways. MDCT clearly maps the relationship of the airway neoplasm to surrounding airways and vasculature, providing critical preoperative information for the surgeon. The intraluminal and extraluminal extent of tumor and presence of postobstructive complications (including air trapping, mucous plugging, atelectasis, and pneumonia) are readily demonstrated on MDCT (Figure 2.9). By detecting the presence of lymphadenopathy and distant metastases, MDCT facilitates accurate staging of the disease and aids in guiding biopsy procedures.

MDCT imaging can determine the amenability of airway neoplasms for complete surgical resection. The approach, type, and extent of surgical resection, including the need for prosthetic airway reconstruction and adjuvant therapy, can be anticipated based on MDCT imaging findings. For those patients who are deemed to be nonsurgical candidates, MDCT can assess the patency of the airways distal to the neoplasm and determine suitability of the airways for airway stent placement.

Although MDCT is highly sensitive for detecting the presence of central airway neoplasms, only rarely do MDCT imaging features allow for an exact diagnosis. Certain MDCT imaging characteristics, however, do enable classification of a neoplasm as benign or malignant.

Benign neoplasms typically are small in size, measuring 2 cm or less in diameter, and appear as round, polypoid, or sessile, focal intraluminal masses. These lesions are well

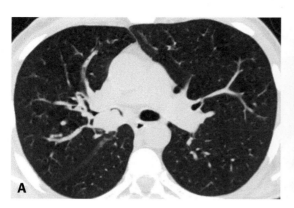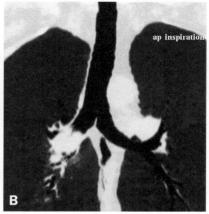

Figure 2.10 Squamous cell carcinoma. **(A)** Axial, noncontrast MDCT image demonstrates a lobulated mass with ill-defined borders within the proximal right main stem bronchus causing near complete occlusion. **(B)** Coronal minimal intensity projection image more clearly displays the size and location of this endobronchial mass with extraluminal extension.

circumscribed and smoothly marginated without evidence of mediastinal invasion or extraluminal extension.

In contrast, malignant airway neoplasms are usually larger in size, often measuring 2–4 cm in diameter. These lesions are often flat or lobulated masses, and their margins are irregular or poorly defined (Figure 2.10). Extramural extension and mediastinal invasion may be present. In 10 percent of malignant airway neoplasms, circumferential airway wall thickening and associated luminal narrowing may be present, findings that are highly characteristic of malignancy. Lymphadenopathy is more commonly seen in cases of malignancy; however, reactive lymphadenopathy may be present in both benign and malignant tumors that are complicated by postobstruction pneumonia. Thus, biopsy of enlarged lymph nodes is necessary for accurate staging purposes.

Although most airway neoplasms are soft tissue in attenuation (a nonspecific finding), in some cases, the MDCT density of an airway lesion can enable a specific diagnosis. MDCT is remarkably sensitive and specific in the detection of fat, and the identification of fat within an airway neoplasm indicates a benign etiology. The most common fat-containing airway tumors include lipomas and hamartomas. The presence of calcification within an airway neoplasm can be seen both in carcinoids and in cartilaginous tumors, including chondroma, chondroblastoma, and chondrosarcoma. Recognition of both fat and calcification within an airway tumor is virtually diagnostic for a hamartoma. MDCT enhancement characteristics may also further enable a diagnosis. For example, carcinoid tumors characteristically demonstrate marked homogenous enhancement after the administration of intravenous contrast (Figure 2.9).

Congenital Airway Disorders

MDCT imaging is an excellent, noninvasive technique for evaluating congenital airway abnormalities, particularly in young children in whom bronchoscopy is often avoided because of its invasive nature and need for general anesthesia. Recently, Heyer and colleagues

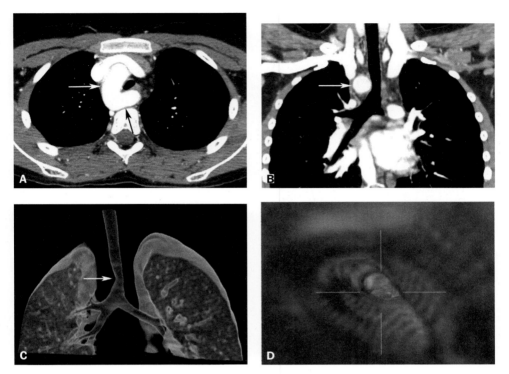

Figure 2.11 Right aortic arch with aberrant left subclavian artery. **(A)** Axial, contrast-enhanced MDCT image shows a right aortic arch (*white arrow*) with aberrant left subclavian artery (*black arrow*) coursing posteriorly to the trachea, causing airway luminal narrowing. **(B)** Coronal multiplanar reformatted image shows the origin of the aberrant left subclavian artery (*arrow*) causing extrinsic lateral compression on the trachea. External **(C)** and internal **(D)** 3D renderings of the trachea clearly depict extent and length of extrinsic airway compression and luminal narrowing (*arrow*). *Courtesy of Edward Lee, MD.*

described low-dose MDCT techniques that substantially limit the radiation dose to children but remain 87 percent sensitive for diagnosing central airway abnormalities with a positive predictive value of 97 percent. MDCT can easily elucidate the cause of congenital airway stenoses, which may be due to either an intrinsic cause such as complete tracheal rings, or an extrinsic cause, such as compression resulting from vascular rings, pulmonary slings, or other aberrant or abnormal mediastinal vasculature (Figure 2.11). Congenital airway anomalies, including tracheoesophageal fistulas, tracheal and bronchial hypoplasia or agenesis, supernumerary or accessory airways, and anomalous airway branching, can be clearly illustrated, particularly with multiplanar and 3D reformation techniques.

Tracheobronchomalacia: Use of Dynamic Expiratory MDCT
Tracheobronchomalacia is a condition defined by excessive collapse of the central airways during expiration due to weakness of the airway walls and supporting cartilage. Tracheobronchomalacia is believed to be a widely underdiagnosed condition, as this disease escapes detection on routine end-inspiratory MDCT imaging.

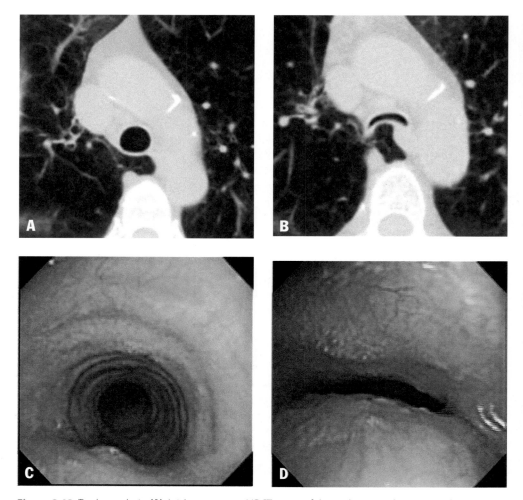

Figure 2.12 Tracheomalacia. **(A)** Axial, noncontrast MDCT image of the trachea at end inspiration shows normal configuration of the airway. **(B)** Axial, noncontrast MDCT image of the trachea obtained at the same level as in **(A)** but during dynamic expiration demonstrates marked collapse of the airway lumen with a "frown-like" appearance, consistent with severe malacia. Conventional bronchoscopic images on inspiration **(C)** and expiration **(D)** confirm MDCT findings.

Paired end-inspiratory, dynamic expiratory MDCT imaging of the central airways has been shown to be a highly sensitive method for detecting excessive airway collapse in patients with bronchoscopically proven tracheobronchomalacia. Historically, the diagnosis of airway malacia on MDCT is established when the cross-sectional area of the airway lumen collapses more than 50 percent on dynamic expiration when compared with end inspiration (Figure 2.12). Recently, however, studies of healthy volunteers with normal pulmonary function have reported mean levels of expiratory collapse in the trachea, right and left main bronchi of 54, 67, and 61 percent, respectively. Moreover, in a minority of healthy individuals, the bronchus intermedius may show complete expiratory collapse. Although future studies are necessary to precisely determine a more rigorous threshold for diagnosing tracheobronchomalacia, it is likely that such a threshold will be defined as at least >70 percent expiratory collapse. In the meantime, in order to avoid over diagnosis of this condition, the identification of excessive airway collapse on CT or bronchoscopy should be closely correlated with clinical symptoms, risk factors, and pulmonary function testing.

Although a diagnosis of tracheobronchomalacia is usually made quantitatively, a characteristic "frown-like" appearance of the airway caused by excessive anterior bowing of the posterior membranous airway wall may be observed in approximately half of patients with this condition (Figure 2.12). From a practical standpoint, this sign can be helpful in identifying tracheobronchomalacia when patients inadvertently breathe during routine CT studies. Ideally, however, the diagnosis should be confirmed on a dedicated dynamic expiratory CT study. MDCT imaging during dynamic expiration, or forceful exhalation, is preferable to imaging at end expiration as a greater degree of collapse is elicited with the former technique in patients with airway malacia. The dynamic expiratory technique has been shown to have a high sensitivity (97 percent) for detecting tracheobronchomalacia in comparison with the "gold standard" of bronchoscopy. Thus, MDCT can be used to screen patients for this condition. Additionally, dynamic expiratory MDCT imaging allows for visualization of air trapping within the lung parenchyma, a finding that is increased in frequency and severity in patients with tracheobronchomalacia in comparison to patients without this condition. After a diagnosis of tracheobronchomalacia has been established, MDCT imaging can facilitate airway stent placement and presurgical planning for tracheoplasty, a novel technique that reinforces the posterior membranous wall with a Marlex graft (Figure 2.13). This promising treatment is reserved for patients with severely symptomatic tracheobronchomalacia often following a successful short-term trial of silicone stenting. Sagittal 2D reformation images along the axis of the trachea, and 3D external reconstructions are particularly useful in delineating the longitudinal extent and severity of airway collapse during dynamic expiration (Figures 2.14 and 2.15).

Multidetector Computed Tomography Imaging: Complementary Role to Bronchoscopy

Although MDCT can never completely supplant conventional bronchoscopy, we emphasize that crucial supplementary information can be gleaned from MDCT imaging both preprocedurally and postprocedurally. In certain cases, MDCT may obviate the need for diagnostic bronchoscopy, thus allowing the bronchoscopist to proceed directly to a therapeutic bronchoscopic procedure. Many endobronchial procedures including laser photocoagulation, brachytherapy, endobronchial cryotherapy, and endobronchial stent placement can be facilitated with MDCT image guidance. Transbronchial biopsies, in particular, can benefit from both virtual and real-time image guidance provided by MDCT. Virtual bronchoscopy in combination with MDCT axial and 2D reformation images can help the pulmonologist determine the ideal location for transbronchial biopsy, particularly for those endobronchially invisible lesions that do not cause mucosal or airway distortion. Additionally, virtual bronchoscopy can help plan the optimal course for passage of bronchoscopic instruments into lesions lying beyond the optic limits of a conventional bronchoscope. As opposed to virtual techniques, CT fluoroscopy can provide real-time, active guidance of transbronchial biopsies. With CT fluoroscopy, the position of the needle can be easily confirmed or simply adjusted.

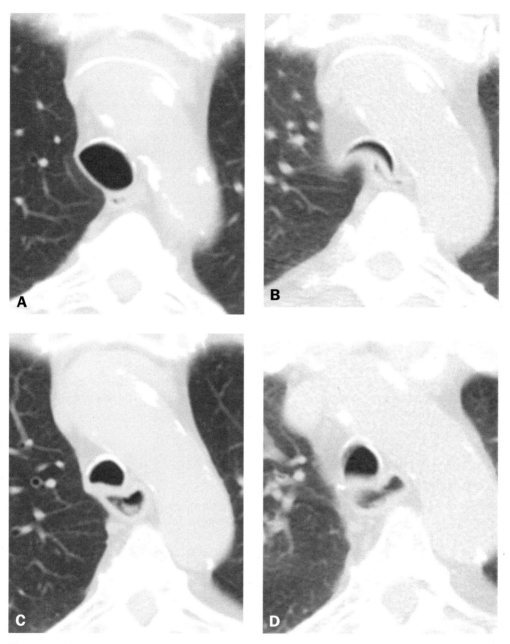

Figure 2.13 Pre- and posttracheoplasty surgery. Axial noncontrast MDCT images of the trachea at the level of the aortic arch prior to surgery at end inspiration **(A)** and during dynamic expiration **(B)** show severe collapse of the trachea consistent with tracheomalacia. Post-tracheoplasty, axial noncontrast MDCT images at end inspiration **(C)** and during dynamic expiration **(D)** demonstrate resolution of tracheomalacia.

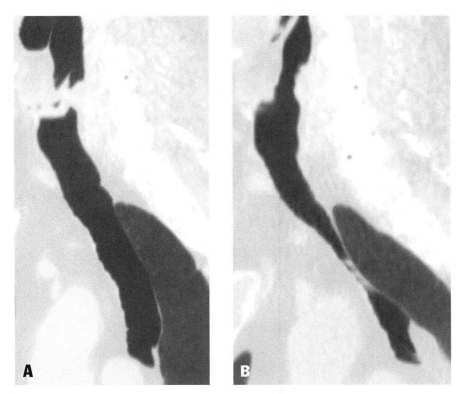

Figure 2.14 Tracheomalacia. **(A)** Sagittal minimal intensity projection image at end inspiration demonstrates a normal appearance of the trachea. **(B)** On dynamic expiration, sagittal minimal intensity projection image not only shows severe anteroposterior collapse of the intrathoracic trachea, but also clearly delineates the craniocaudal extent of malacia.

Prestent and Poststent Evaluation

In addition to providing both virtual and real-time guidance for transbronchial biopsies, MDCT can also provide important preprocedural and postprocedural information for endobronchial stent placement. Prior to stent placement, MDCT serves to elucidate the anatomy, pathology, severity, and extent of airway obstruction. Imaging information can help identify the source of airway obstruction as being caused by extraluminal compression, intraluminal disease, or intrinsic disease, such as from tracheobronchomalacia. Additionally, MDCT can detail distal airway anatomy not visualized with conventional bronchoscopy. Importantly, MDCT imaging findings can help decide which patients are amenable to surgical resection and which patients are candidates for palliative options such as airway stenting. For those patients suitable for endobronchial stenting, MDCT findings can help select the type, endoluminal size, and length of stent needed.

Although flexible bronchoscopy is the conventional method of follow-up after stent placement, MDCT is ideally suited to image the airways after endobronchial stenting. All endo-bronchial stents, whether silicone or metallic, create minimal artifacts on MDCT, and therefore are well visualized on MDCT imaging. The precise location, shape, and patency of

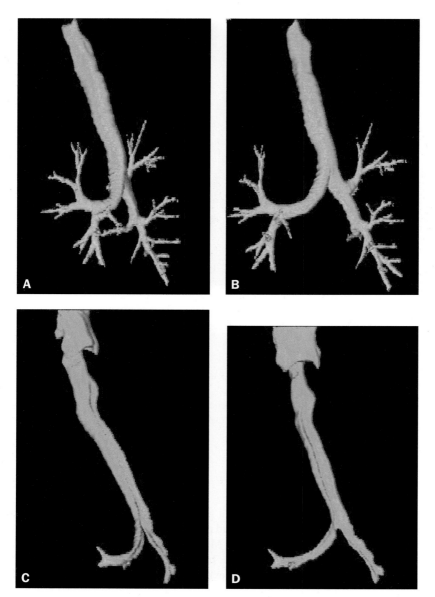

Figure 2.15 Tracheobronchomalacia. Sagittal **(A)** and oblique **(B)** 3D external reconstructions of the central airways at end inspiration demonstrate normal trachea and bronchi. Sagittal **(C)** and oblique **(D)** 3D external reconstruction images of the central airways during dynamic expiration show diffuse tracheobronchomalacia with pruned appearance of the segmental bronchi due to severe luminal collapse.

the stent as well as its relationship to adjacent airways can be clearly delineated with MDCT and multiplanar imaging. Furthermore, MDCT is highly accurate in detecting stent complications, including malpositioning, migration, fracture, size discrepancy between stent and airway, development of excessive in-stent granulation tissue, mucoid impaction, infection,

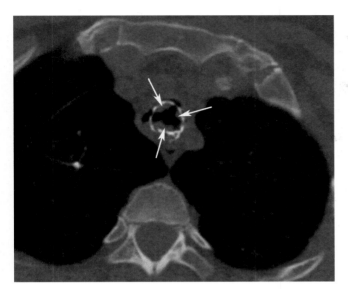

Figure 2.16 Size discrepancy between tracheal stent and airway lumen. Axial noncontrast MDCT image of the trachea demonstrates tracheal lumen to be larger than the caliber of the tracheal stent. Additionally, polypoid soft-tissue opacities (*arrows*) projecting into the lumen of the stent are compatible with granulation tissue.

external airway stent compression with continued stenosis, and tumor ingrowth/local recurrence of malignancy (Figure 2.16). When compared with bronchoscopy, MDCT with 2D multiplanar and 3D reconstruction techniques has been shown to be 88 percent to 100 percent sensitive and 100 percent specific in identifying stent complications. Indeed, MDCT can serve as a noninvasive, highly accurate method for stent surveillance.

Summary

MDCT imaging with 2D multiplanar reformation and 3D reconstruction techniques allows for rapid, noninvasive, and accurate assessment of the tracheobronchial tree. A variety of pathologic processes involving the airways – including airway stenoses, central airway neoplasms, and congenital airway disorders – can be clearly illustrated in a visually accessible manner to the bronchoscopist, thereby providing key information needed for preprocedural planning. The use of dynamic expiratory imaging in conjunction with standard end-inspiratory MDCT imaging is a sensitive technique for the diagnosis of tracheobronchomalacia. MDCT plays an important complementary role to bronchoscopy by providing critical preprocedural and postprocedural information. MDCT can enhance guidance of bronchoscopic procedures, including sampling of lesions invisible on conventional bronchoscopy. Finally, MDCT is emerging as a primary, noninvasive method for the surveillance of the airways after bronchoscopic interventions, particularly after endoluminal stent placement.

Further Readings

Baroni RH, Feller-Kopman D, Nishino M, Hatabu H, Loring SH, Ernst A, Boiselle PM. Tracheobronchomalacia: comparison between end-expiratory and dynamic expiratory CT for evaluation of central airway collapse. *Radiology*. 2005;235:635–641.

Boiselle PM, Lee KS, Ernst A. Multidetector CT of the central airways. *J Thorac Imaging*. 2005;20: 186–195.

Boiselle PM, O'Donnell CR, Bankier AA, et al. Tracheal collapsibility in healthy volunteers during forced expiration: assessment with multidetector CT. *Radiology*. 2009;252:255–262.

Boiselle PM, Feller-Kopman D, Ashiku S, Weeks D, Ernst A. Tracheobronchomalacia: evolving role of dynamic multislice helical CT. *Radiol Clin North Am*. 2003;41:627–636.

Gilkeson RC, Ciancibello LM, Hejal RB, Montenegro HD, Lange P. Tracheobronchomalacia: dynamic airway evaluation with multidetector CT. *AJR Am J Roentgenol*. 2001;176:205–210.

Godoy MCB, Saldana DA, Rao PP, Vlahos I, Naidich DP, Benveniste MF, Erasmus JJ, Marom EM, Ost D. Multidetector CT evaluation of airway stents: what the radiologist should know. *Radiographics*. 2014;34:7;1793–1806.

Heyer CM, Nuesslein TG, Jung D, Peters SA, Lemburg SP, Rieger CH, Nicolas V. Tracheobronchial anomalies and stenoses: detection with low-dose multidetector CT with virtual tracheobronchoscopy–comparison with flexible tracheobronchoscopy. *Radiology*. 2007;242: 542–549.

Hoppe H, Dinkel HP, Walder B, von Allmen G, Gugger M, Vock P. Grading airway stenosis down to the segmental level using virtual bronchoscopy. *Chest*. 2004;125:704–711.

Lee KS, Lunn W, Feller-Kopman D, Ernst A, Hatabu H, Boiselle PM. Multislice CT evaluation of airway stents. *J Thorac Imaging*. 2005;20:81–88.

Lee KS, Sun MR, Ernst A, Feller-Kopman D, Majid A, Boiselle PM. Comparison of dynamic expiratory CT with bronchoscopy for diagnosing airway malacia: a pilot evaluation. *Chest*. 2007; 131:758–764.

Litmanovich D, O'Donnell CR, Bankier AA, et al. Bronchial collapsibility at forced expiration in healthy volunteers: assessment with multidetector CT. *Radiology*. 2010;257:560–567.

McCarthy MJ, Rosado-de-Christenson ML. Tumors of the trachea. *J Thorac Imaging*. 1995;10: 180–198.

Quint LE, Whyte RI, Kazerooni EA, Martinez FJ, Cascade PN, Lynch JP Orringer MB, Brunsting LA 3rd, Deeb GM. Stenosis of the central airways: evaluation by using helical CT with multiplanar reconstructions. *Radiology*. 1995;194:871–877.

Remy-Jardin M, Remy J, Artaud D, Fribourg M, Duhamel A. Volume rendering of the tracheobronchial tree: clinical evaluation of bronchographic images. *Radiology*. 1998;208:761–770.

Ridge CA, O'Donnell CR, Lee EY, et al. Tracheobronchomalacia: current concepts and controversies. *J Thorac Imaging*. 2011;26:278–289.

Siegel MJ. Multiplanar and three-dimensional multi-detector row CT of thoracic vessels and airways in the pediatric population. *Radiology*. 2003;229:641–650.

Chapter 3

The Larynx

Daniel C. Chelius, Jr. and William W. Lunn

The human voice is the organ of the soul.
Henry Wadsworth Longfellow

Introduction

The larynx is a complex constricting and dilating gateway to the trachea. The three primary functions of the larynx are (1) protection of the airway, (2) respiration, and (3) phonation. Laryngeal closure also allows the patient to build up intra-thoracic pressure (the Valsalva maneuver) prior to coughing. It is essential for physicians performing diagnostic or treatment procedures in or through the upper aerodigestive tract to be familiar with the larynx. The purpose of this chapter is twofold: (1) to discuss laryngeal anatomy and function, and (2) to suggest an approach to laryngeal examination.

Anatomy

Although it sits on top of the trachea, the larynx is suspended from the sternum, clavicles, skull base, mandible, and anterior vertebral column by a group of extrinsic muscles. Its skeleton is a series of cartilages held together by ligaments, elastic membranes, and the intrinsic laryngeal muscles.

Cartilages

The cricoid cartilage forms the base of the larynx. Although the larynx is a tubular structure, the cricoid is the only complete cartilaginous ring in the laryngeal skeleton. Thus, injury to the larynx in the region of the cricoid ring from trauma, tumor, or iatrogenic causes may quickly lead to laryngeal collapse and airway obstruction. The cricoid has a signet ring shape and is much taller posteriorly (20–30 mm) than anteriorly (5–7 mm). While the anterior cricoid is palpable below the thyroid cartilage during neck examination, the posterior cricoid rises past the inferior level of the thyroid cartilage (Figure 3.1).

Posteriorly, the cricoid supports the arytenoids: paired, lightweight pyramid-shaped cartilages that are the mobile posterior attachment point for the vocal cords (Figure 3.2). The cricoarytenoid articulation is a synovial joint that allows the arytenoids to move sideways as well as to slide downward toward the midline. In combination, these movements create the vocal cord abduction (outward movement away from midline) and adduction (inward movement towards midline) essential for proper laryngeal function. Like any other synovial joint, the cricoarytenoid joint is subject to a wide spectrum of pathology including arthritis (infectious or inflammatory), ankylosis (fixation), and dislocation, which can impede vocal

Figure 3.1 The larynx in cross section.

Epiglottis

Thyroid Cartilage

Vocal Fold

Arytenoid Cartilage

Cricoid Cartilage

Proximal Trachea

Cut surfaces are lined

cord mobility. The corniculate cartilages sit atop the arytenoids and project posteromedially. During vocal cord adduction, they approach each other in the midline and exert laterally directed elastic recoil on the posterior vocal cords. The cuneiform cartilages are suspended in the aryepiglottic fold and are often visible as raised white masses during endoscopy, sometimes mistaken for malignancy or a submucosal cyst.

The thyroid cartilage is the largest and most prominent laryngeal cartilage. It is shaped like a shield and appropriately named (*thyrus* = shield, Greek) as it protects the internal anatomy of the larynx. The thyroid cartilage has paired superior and inferior horns, or cornu. The superior cornu have ligamentous attachments to the hyoid above, an important part of the laryngeal suspension. The inferior cornu articulate with the lateral cricoid cartilage. This cricothyroid joint is also a synovial joint that allows anteriorposterior rocking of the thyroid cartilage on the cricoid; therefore, it is also susceptible to the pathologies mentioned earlier.

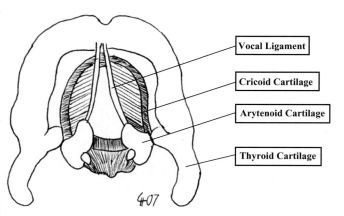

Figure 3.2 The larynx viewed from above.

Vocal Ligament

Cricoid Cartilage

Arytenoid Cartilage

Thyroid Cartilage

The epiglottis contains the leaf-shaped epiglottic cartilage that is suspended anteriorly from the hyoid and inferiorly from the thyroid by a series of ligaments. As the larynx tips anterosuperiorly during swallowing, the epiglottic base is pushed against the tongue base causing the epiglottis to fold over the laryngeal inlet. Although the hyoid is not typically considered part of the larynx, it is intimately associated with the superior cartilages and important in the laryngeal suspension. The hyoid, thyroid, cricoid, and arytenoids are composed of hyaline cartilage and progressively ossify. The hyoid is completely ossified by age two; the thyroid begins ossifying in the early twenties, and the cricoid and arytenoids follow shortly thereafter.

Membranes

There are two important submucosal elastic membranes in the larynx: the quadrangular membrane superiorly and the conus elasticus inferiorly. The quadrangular membrane joins the lateral epiglottis, the arytenoids, and corniculate cartilages. The inferior border joins the vestibular ligament above the vocal fold to form the "false vocal cord" while the superior border and its membranous covering form the aryepiglottic fold. The conus elasticus joins the superior border of the cricoid to the thyroid and arytenoid cartilages. The superior edge of the conus elasticus runs between the midline posterior thyroid cartilage (anterior commissure) and the vocal process of the arytenoids. This free edge is the vocal ligament, the elastic component of the true vocal cord.

Muscles

The intrinsic muscles of the larynx cause the configuration changes in the laryngeal cartilages that open or close and loosen or tighten the vocal cords. The paired thyroarytenoid, lateral cricoarytenoid, and unpaired interartenoid muscles adduct the vocal cords while the paired posterior cricoarytenoid muscles are the only abductors. The paired cricothyroid muscles tip the thyroid cartilage anteriorly on the cricoid, tightening the vocal cords further.

The extrinsic muscles of the larynx suspend it in the soft tissues of the neck. The laryngeal elevators raise and anteriorly displace the larynx during swallowing to prevent aspiration. These include the stylohyoid, digastric, and stylopharyngeus from the skull base and the geniohyoid and mylohyoid from the mandible. The elevating forces exerted on the hyoid are transmitted to the larynx by the thyrohyoid muscle and ligaments. The laryngeal depressors displace the larynx downward during inspiration and include the remaining strap muscles – omohyoid, sternohyoid, and sternothyroid. The esophageal constrictors and cricopharyngeus insert on the posterior larynx and are critical to the swallowing reflex.

Mucosa

The larynx is lined by two different types of mucosa. The free edges of the true vocal cords, upper edges of the aryepiglottic folds and superior epiglottis are covered in stratified squamous epithelium while the remainder of the larynx is covered in pseudo-stratified ciliated columnar respiratory epithelium. The mucosa is a continuous sheet as it wraps over top of the epiglottis and reflects onto the tongue base, forming the vallecula. A layer of loose connective tissue is immediately deep to the mucosa in the bulk of the larynx. However, this layer of connective tissue is absent on the laryngeal (posterior) surface of the epiglottis which accounts for the marked anterior epiglottic swelling that can be seen in epiglottitis or supraglottitis.

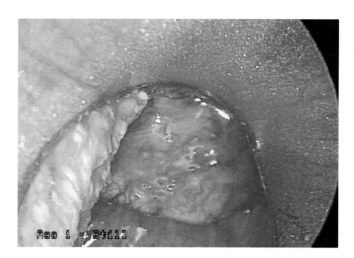

Figure 3.3 The tongue base, epiglottis, and vallecula.

The submucosal layers of the vocal cord are completely distinct from the remainder of the larynx, and deserve special attention. The vocal cord consists of three main layers: the stratified squamous cover, the trilamellar lamina propria, and the vocalis muscle. The superficial layer of the lamina propria is a very loose connective tissue that has the consistency of a soft gelatin. This is the primary layer in which vibration during phonation occurs and is also the layer most likely to become filled with edematous fluid due to its loose configuration. The intermediate and deep layers of the lamina propria consist of elastic and collagen fibers, respectively. These layers form the vocal ligament, and are the termination of the conus elasticus.

Innervation

The superior and inferior laryngeal nerves arise from the vagus nerve to innervate the intrinsic muscles and mucosa of the larynx. The superior nerve branches off at the nodose ganglion, passes deep to the carotid artery, runs lateral to the larynx in the submucosa of the piriform sinus, and then divides into internal and external branches. The internal branch pierces the thyrohyoid membrane with the superior laryngeal artery to give sensory and secretory innervation to the laryngeal mucosa above the true vocal cords. The external branch runs lateral to the thyroid cartilage to innervate the cricothyroid muscle. The inferior laryngeal nerve is the termination of the recurrent laryngeal nerve. The recurrent laryngeal branches off the vagus in the chest and wraps around the subclavian artery on the right and the aortic arch on the left before ascending in the tracheoesophageal groove. The inferior nerve pierces the cricothyroid membrane and provides motor innervation to all of the intrinsic muscles except the cricothyroid. The recurrent laryngeal nerve is not well organized internally so that when the nerve is divided, reanastamosis does not typically restore normal motor function.

Endoscopic Landmarks

From a superior vantage point during endoscopic examination of the larynx, there are a number of important landmarks to consider. Starting anteriorly, the tongue base, vallecula, and epiglottis can be easily appreciated in most patients (Figure 3.3). In order to fully visualize

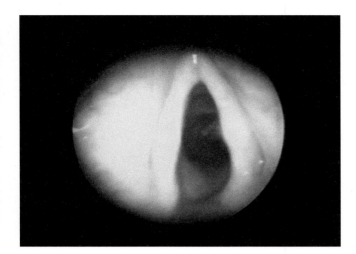

Figure 3.4 The normal larynx.

these structures, it may be necessary for the patient to slightly protrude the tongue if they suffer from "pharyngeal crowding" or obesity. Moving posterior and inferior, the aryepiglottic folds lead down to the arytenoids with bumps in the mucosa representing the underlying cuneiform and corniculate cartilages. The laryngeal surface of the epiglottis leads down to the anterior commissure at the level of the true vocal cords (Figure 3.4). However, above the true vocal cords is the vestibule, superiorly bound by the false vocal cords (Figure 3.5). The true vocal cords can be divided into the more anterior portion, which are primarily responsible for the vibration leading to phonation, and the posterior portion. The posterior intercartilaginous area is the site of articulation of the vocal cord with the vocal process of the arytenoid cartilage. The postcricoid space lies behind the larynx and the piriform sinuses lie laterally. The piriforms are pyramid-shaped with the bases superior at the level of the laryngeal inlet and the apices at the inlet of the esophagus. The piriform apices are not always visible during flexible endoscopic examination. The examiner may ask the patient to puff their cheeks out

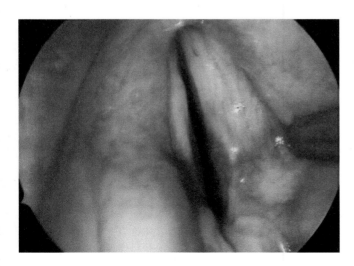

Figure 3.5 The true and false cords, with a probe in the vestibule.

Table 3.1 Systematic Laryngeal Examination

Anatomic Landmarks	Exam Parameters (ACCMME)
Tongue Base	Airway
Vallecula	Contour
Epiglottis	Color
Aryepiglottic Fold	Mucosa
Posterior Glottis	Mobility
False Vocal Cords	Edema
Vestibule	
True Vocal Cords	
Anterior Commissure	
Subglottis	
Piriform Sinuses	
Posterior and Lateral Pharyngeal Walls	

in order to better visualize the piriforms during endoscopy. The subglottic larynx is the area below the true cords and is very vulnerable to injury as discussed earlier.

Endoscopic Examination

It is essential for the novice and the expert alike to develop a consistent routine for laryngeal examination in order to minimize missed findings. A standard vocabulary for describing laryngeal findings will facilitate accurate and efficient communication between specialists. We have found it useful to systematically move through anatomic landmarks while considering a specific set of examination parameters parameters (Table 3.1). The mnemonic ACCMME outlines a helpful exam system.

The first and most critical aspect of laryngeal examination is ensuring a widely patent airway. Many decisions about subsequent management hinge on the examiner's description of the airway stability. The airway may be obstructed at the larynx from varied etiologies. Each laryngeal exam should include a simple subjective characterization of the airway as widely patent, patent, narrowed, marginal, or critical.

The laryngeal mucosa is typically pink with the exception of the true vocal cords which should be pearly white. In either of these locations, the color should be homogenous. Variability in color may be an early sign of pathology. For example, erythema typically indicates hypervascularity or inflammation that may be a sign of upper respiratory infection, posttussive laryngitis, early cancer, or acid reflux. On the other hand, chronic acid reflux causes a gray discoloration and heaping up of the interarytenoid mucosa known as pachydermia. The true vocal cords may assume a dusky gray color in smokers. Whitish discoloration, also known as leukoplakia, is an early sign of neoplasia. Submucosal vascular lesions may give the mucosa a purple or bluish hue. Overall laryngeal color and the specific location of color abnormalities should be recorded.

Detecting alterations in the contour or position of laryngeal structures requires extensive experience with the normal laryngeal exam. Effacement of normal pharyngeal or laryngeal spaces such as the vallecula, piriform sinuses, and vestibule may indicate a submucosal

Table 3.2 Common Laryngeal Mucosal Abnormalities

Lesion	Location	Description
Retention Cyst	Vallecula, vestibule, undersurface of vocal cord	Unilateral, smooth, filled with clear or straw colored fluid
Epidermoid Cyst	Medial edge of vocal cord	Unilateral, submucosal, smooth, white
Vocal Cord Nodule	Junction of anterior and middle thirds of cords	Paired; Initially: smooth, soft, red; Mature: hard, white, fibrotic
Vocal Cord Polyps	Medial edge of vocal cord	Unilateral, pedunculated, fusiform, or diffuse
Contact Ulcer	Posterior vocal process of arytenoid	Bilateral, red, ulcerated
Intubation Granuloma	Posterior vocal process of arytenoid	Unilateral, red, large, and pedunculated
Papilloma	Vocal cords or vestibule	Heaped up, warty appearance, pink or red, multifocal
Hemangioma	Variable	Purple or blue, submucosal
Squamous Cell Carcinoma	Variable	Initially: flat whitish plaque with irregular borders; Mature: large, irregular, white or red, ulcerated

mass, abscess, hematoma, or infiltrative process. More subtle contour changes like asymmetric twisting or tilting of structures may also indicate an infiltrative process. Abnormally sized or absent laryngeal landmarks can also be pathologic. Vallecular effacement may be a surrogate marker for an enlarged tongue base, a contributing factor in obstructive sleep apnea. Neurologic lesions can also result in subtle contour changes. Damage to the external branch of the superior laryngeal nerve causes the larynx to rotate away from the side with the lesion while damage to the inferior laryngeal nerve can result in a malpositioned vocal cord. Contour irregularities can be difficult to describe. The description can include position relative to nearby normal landmarks or to the normal larynx as a reference.

The laryngeal mucosa is susceptible to the same diseases as any other similar epithelium including carcinoma, bacterial/fungal/viral infections, and inflammatory or autoimmune ulcerations. Because the vocal cords are repeatedly forced together for phonation, coughing, and airway protection, the vocal cord mucosa is prone to trauma-related conditions such as granulomas and contact ulcerations. This is especially true when a patient inappropriately strains the vocal cords through vocal abuse. Traumatic hemorrhage into the vocal cord can occur with such prolonged abuse or with acute severe trauma from yelling or forceful singing. Such a hemorrhage can eventually transform into a vocal cord nodule. Finally, direct trauma to the vocal cords from extrinsic forces such as traumatic intubation or prolonged intubation can result in similar contact-related pathologies. Table 3.2 lists some common mucosal abnormalities with clues to differential diagnosis. Figures 3.6–3.10 provide examples of some of the lesions described in Table 3.2.

All critical laryngeal functions rely on normal laryngeal mobility. Examining the laryngeal mobility requires more than simply detecting vocal cord paralysis. It involves assessing the quality of vocal cord movement and picking up subtle clues about underlying pathology not necessarily visible through the scope. The voice is a sensitive indicator of appropriate vocal fold movement, so this part of the exam begins when first encountering a patient. Many examiners report any abnormal voice as "hoarse." There are many characteristics of an abnormal voice that are more informative than such a catch-all phrase. A voice may be high or low, soft or loud, weak or powerful, breathy or clear, sharp or dull, sonorous or thin, resonant or

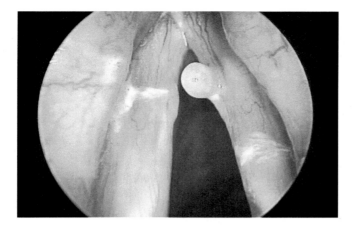

Figure 3.6 TVC Polyp: A smooth, pink, pedunculated lesion of the anterior right vocal cord.

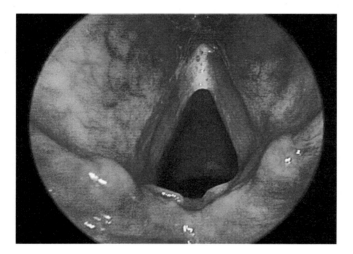

Figure 3.7 TVC Reflux: Laryngeal edema with heaped up mucosa and ulceration over the arytenoids and interarytenoid space.

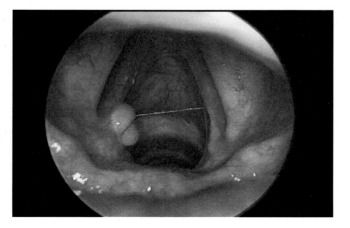

Figure 3.8 TVC Granuloma: Smooth white lesion over the left vocal process.

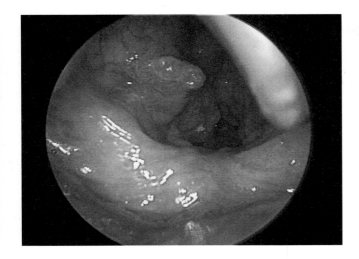

Figure 3.9 TVC Papillomas: Heaped up, smooth, warty lesions disturbing the normal vocal cord contours. Involves the supraglottis, glottis, and subglottis.

falsetto, periodic or raw and harsh, relaxed or tense and strained. Various pathologies have typical vocal alterations that essentially fall within this set of descriptors. In addition to laryngeal mobility, inadequate breath support from diseased lower airways can also alter the voice and should be considered as well.

The term stridor is used to describe loud upper airway sounds that are generated by turbulent airflow. When present, the examiner should note if stridor occurs during inspiration, expiration, or both. While stridor often results from pathology in the larynx, it can also be produced by disease in the upper trachea.

The majority of laryngeal mobility disorders can be diagnosed from history and laryngoscopy with a flexible scope. To assess vocal cord movement, the glottis is examined while the patient phonates. Sustained long vowel sounds (ē) at various pitches are best for assessing gross vocal cord movement, while short phrases ("every," "each," "Harry likes hamburgers") are best for assessing coordination. When an abnormality in vocal cord movement is detected, asking the patient to count as high as possible on one breath gives a baseline idea of how much the abnormality affects breath control.

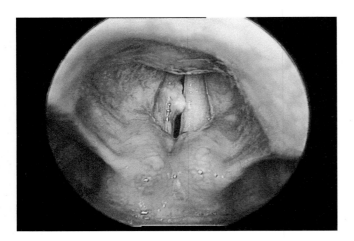

Figure 3.10 TVC Cancer: Irregular white lesion of the left vocal cord.

The vocal cords rest in the abducted position approximately 25° from the midline and move symmetrically toward the midline during phonation. A completely immobile vocal cord may be paralyzed by deinnervation, fixed by some infiltrative process, or fixed due to cricoarytenoid joint disease. The paralyzed cord will typically rest in the midline with a bowed appearance whereas the fixed cord may be in any position, bowed or taut, depending on the underlying pathology. In either case, the contralateral vocal fold may cross the midline, making contact with the immobile cord and preserving better laryngeal function than would be expected. Additionally, the false vocal folds may be voluntarily or involuntarily used to phonate, especially in the case of a unilateral vocal cord paralysis. This is called plicae ventricularis, and it can make assessment of the vocal cord mobility much more difficult. Frequently, laryngeal examination reveals a problem with vocal cord movement less severe than outright immobility. This can be described as weakness or paresis.

Finally, the larynx should be carefully examined for edema which may be mild in the case of acid reflux or possibly life-threatening in the cases of supraglottitis or angioedema. Vocal cord edema (Reinke's edema) is most frequently seen in women with hypothyroidism or smokers. However, this is usually not a life-threatening situation and can be managed medically. Careful note should be made of the exact laryngeal structures that are edematous so that improvement or worsening can be documented with serial exams.

Conclusion

The larynx is a complex and elegant organ; it is not something to "get past in order to do the bronchoscopy." Many decisions about airway management hinge on the status of the larynx. A proper understanding of laryngeal anatomy and function is necessary for one to become an expert bronchoscopist.

Further Readings

Hirano M and Kiminori S. *Histological Color Atlas of the Human Larynx*. San Francisco: Singular Publishing Group, Inc., 1993.

Hurley Robert. *The Larynx: A Multidisciplinary Approach*, 2nd Ed. St. Louis: Mosby, 1996.

Lehmann W, Pidoux JM, and Widmann JJ. *Larynx: Microlaryngoscopy and Histopathology*. Cadempino, Switzerland: Inpharzam SA, 1981.

Sasaki CT and Kim TH. "Anatomy and physiology of the larynx." *Ballenger's Otorhinolaryngology Head and Neck Surgery*, 16th Ed. Ontario: BC Decker Inc. 2003;1090–1109.

Yanagisawa E. *Color Atlas of Diagnostic Endoscopy in Otorhinolaryngology*. New York: Igaku-Shoin Medical Publishers, 1997.

Airway Anatomy for the Bronchoscopist

Shana Hill, Rani Kumaran, Arthur Sung, and Armin Ernst

Introduction

Bronchoscopy is a diagnostic and therapeutic procedure that permits direct visualization of normal and pathological alterations of the upper and lower airways. Expert knowledge of airway anatomy is a prerequisite for successful performance of the procedure. The major advantages of the flexible bronchoscope (FB) include the ability to insert it nasally, orally, or through a tracheostomy stoma to visualize apical segments of upper lobes as well as segmental and subsegmental bronchi in all lobes. This chapter focuses on identification of normal anatomy, landmarks, and pathologies seen during bronchoscopy of upper airways (from nares to glottis) and lower airways (trachea and conducting bronchi). It will also briefly touch on multidetecter computed tomography as a tool for assessment of airways and diagnosis of disease such as tracheobronchomalacia.

Bronchoscopists commonly refer to airway anatomy according to the Jackson–Huber classification with segmental airway anatomy named according to spatial orientation (i.e., anterior/posterior, superior/inferior, and medial/lateral) (Figure 4.1). Table 4.1 lists the nomenclature accordingly. Many thoracic surgeons prefer to use the Boyden surgical classification, which assigns numbers to the segmental airways (Table 4.1). It is advised that beginning bronchoscopists learn the Jackson–Huber classification first, emphasizing accurate and consistent usage.

The FB is introduced by the bronchoscopist standing either behind the head of the supine patient or facing the patient. The anatomic orientation of airways varies depending on the operator's position. For the purpose of consistency in this chapter, the anatomical orientation is presented with the operator standing behind the supine patient.

Upper Airway

Nasopharynx

The upper airway examination begins with a quick assessment of nasal and oral cavities. When the FB is introduced through the nose, the inferior turbinate is seen laterally and the nasal septum is seen medially. The bronchoscope is then directed posteriorly into the pharynx. When viewing the nasal cavity, the bronchoscopist should assess for septal deviation, hypertrophy of turbinates, presence of polyps, and integrity of mucosa. Serosanguineous nasal drainage with severe crusting may be suggestive of Wegener's granulomatosis. Isolated, large septal perforation with inflamed and crusty edges is highly suggestive of nasal substance abuse. Diffuse nasal crusting or a vasomotor-like appearance to the nasal mucosa can typify sarcoidosis. In appropriate clinical settings, nasal polyps may suggest cause for postnasal

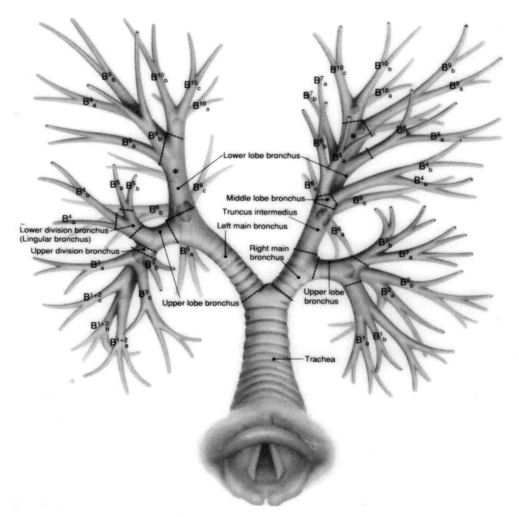

Figure 4.1 Diagrammatic representation of tracheobronchial tree. The authors acknowledge Olympus Company for providing the figure.

drip and reactive airway diseases, such as atopic asthma or vasculitides (e.g., Churg–Strauss syndrome). Nasal tuberculosis may show a red, nodular thickening, with or without ulceration. A rapidly progressive black, necrotic mass of tissue filling the nasal cavity, eroding the nasal septum, and extending through the hard palate characterizes mucormycosis.

Oropharynx and Hypopharynx

When the FB is introduced orally, it passes through the oropharynx and larynx and into the trachea. Beyond the base of the tongue, the bronchoscope is passed through the curvature of the oropharynx, which is bordered superiorly by the soft palate and extends to the tip of the epiglottis. The FB is then directed posterior to the tip of the epiglottis. The three major

Table 4.1 Boyden Surgical Classification / Jackson–Huber Classification

Right Bronchial Tree		Left Bronchial Tree	
RUL		LUL	
B1	Apical	Upper division	
B2	Posterior	B1/2	Apicoposterior
B3	Anterior	B3	Anterior
RML		Lingular	
B4	Lateral	B4	Superior
B5	Medial	B5	Inferior
RLL		LLL	
B6	Superior	B6	Superior
B7	Medial basal	B7/8	Anteromedial
B8	Anterior basal	B9	Lateral basal
B9	Lateral basal	B10	Posterior basal
B10	Posterior		

Note: RUL, right upper lobe; LUL, left upper lobe;
RML, right middle lobe; RLL, right lower lobe; LLL, left lower lobe.

structures in the hypopharynx are the pyriform recess, the postcricoid region, and the posterior pharyngeal wall (Figure 4.2). Tongue size, tooth integrity, and temporomandibular joint mobility are important factors affecting the ease of introduction into the oropharynx. The space between the base of the tongue and the anterior surface of the epiglottis on either side constitutes the vallecula. The valleculae are separated by the median glossoepiglottic fold and bordered laterally on either side by the lateral glossoepiglottic folds. Valleculae are often locations for foreign body entrapment and upper airway obstruction.

Larynx
The bronchoscopist should assess the vocal cords for normal abduction on inspiration and adduction during phonation. Dysfunction of vocal cords can be either functional or organic, as seen in persistent gastroesophageal acid reflux, and can cause significant airway compromise. Paradoxical vocal cord motion is an inappropriate adduction of the true vocal cords throughout the respiratory cycle with the obliteration of glottic aperture except for a posterior diamond-shaped opening.

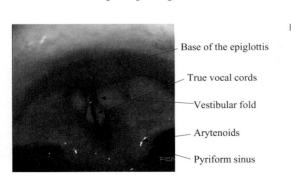

Figure 4.2 Laryngeal anatomy.

Base of the epiglottis

True vocal cords

Vestibular fold

Arytenoids

Pyriform sinus

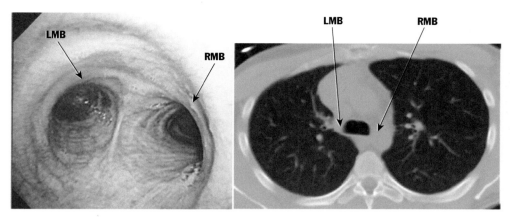

Figure 4.3 Carina with right and left main bronchus. (RMB, right main bronchus; LMB, left main bronchus)

The glossopharyngeal nerve and the vagus nerve supply the motor and sensory pathways for the larynx. The superior laryngeal branch of the vagus nerve (SLN) provides sensory innervation to the glottis, the arytenoids, and the vocal cords. Stimulation of pathways of the SLN, including manipulation of pyriform recess, may result in protective closure of the glottis. Therefore, it is paramount that appropriate topical anesthesia to theses structures be applied prior to proceeding with bronchoscopy.

Lower Airway

Trachea

The lower airway (trachea to conductive bronchi) begins at the cricoid cartilage (at about the level of the sixth cervical vertebra, C6). The adult trachea ranges from 16 to 20 mm in internal diameter and has 18–22 cartilage rings. The trachea tapers slightly and aims posteriorly as it divides at the carina, at the level of fifth thoracic spine to the left and right main stem bronchi. The horseshoe-shaped tracheal cartilage shapes the anterior part of the trachea, whereas the posterior part of the trachea consists of smooth muscles that joins the ends of the tracheal cartilage (Figure 4.3).

Starting at the upper trachea, mucosal integrity should be examined, even when there are no gross endobronchial lesions. The presence of extrinsic tracheal deviation and compression due to paratracheal masses should be noted. Both the anterior cartilaginous and posterior membranous portions of the trachea are sometimes sites for dynamic airway compromise caused by tracheomalacia or excessive dynamic airway collapse. The distal trachea and main carina are important sites for examination because malignant diseases often metastasize to the surrounding mediastinal lymph nodes.

If a lesion is identified, both sides of the lungs should be examined completely before biopsies are taken. The importance of complete surveillance is that unexpected satellite airway pathologies can occur in up to 10 percent of primary bronchogenic carcinomas. After main pathology is visualized or diagnostic procedures are started, the bronchoscopist can become too distracted to return to a thorough and careful examination of the remainder of the airways. Furthermore, when the site of primary pathology is sampled, bleeding can degrade the quality of the FB image, and coughing and oxygen desaturation will limit the time

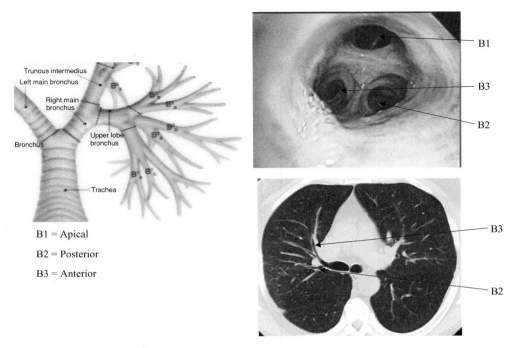

B1 = Apical

B2 = Posterior

B3 = Anterior

Figure 4.4 Right upper lobe.

to complete the procedure. There is also a danger that samples retrieved from a secondary site that appear abnormal and are found to contain malignant cells can actually represent contamination from cells dislodged during earlier examination of a primary malignant site. Such false-positive results may have a devastating effect of overstaging a potentially curable peripheral lesion.

Main Carina

The main carina is a keel-shaped structure oriented anteroposteriorly. On flexible bronchoscopy and chest computed tomography (CT), as seen in Figure 4.3, the main carina is identified as a thin septum separating the right and left main bronchi. It is usually sharp in adults, and its dimensions vary during inhalation and exhalation. The angle of the left main carina is usually 10°–15° higher than the right main carina on CT.

Right Bronchial Tree

The right main bronchus is approximately 1.5 cm in length and has an internal diameter of 10–12 mm. The first branch, the right upper lobe (RUL) bronchus, arises just below the carina, and courses laterally for a distance of 1–2 cm before branching into apical, anterior, and posterior segments as seen in Figure 4.4 in flexible bronchoscopy and chest CT. On a CT scan, the branching point of the RUL bronchus can be identified as a faint curvilinear density marginating the lateral wall of the right main bronchus. The horizontal course of the RUL bronchus with origins of anterior and posterior segments gives the inverted whale tail appearance. These branching points are frequent sites of bronchial disease, including

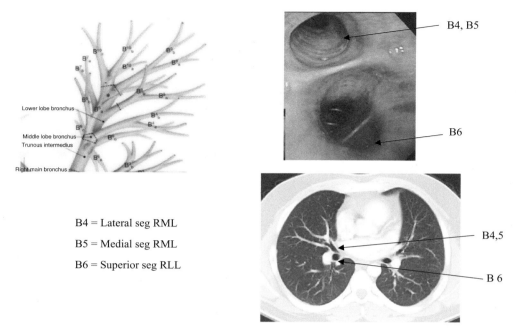

B4 = Lateral seg RML

B5 = Medial seg RML

B6 = Superior seg RLL

Figure 4.5 Right middle lobe and right lower lobe.

carcinoma. On CT imaging, at the level of distal trachea, the apical segment appears as a circular lucency in proximity to pulmonary vessels. Both anterior and posterior (and their subsegments) can be easily seen.

Beyond the RUL bronchus, the right main bronchus becomes the bronchus intermedius, extends approximately 2–2.5 cm, and divides into right middle lobe and lower lobe bronchi as seen in Figure 4.5 in flexible bronchoscopy and chest CT. In chest CT, the bronchus intermedius is characteristically seen on several adjacent sections. It has an oblique shape and courses directly posterior to the right main pulmonary artery and the right interlobar pulmonary artery inferiorly. A cardiac bronchus, a rare congenital anomaly, can be seen arising from the medial wall of the bronchus intermedius before the origin of the superior segmental branch of the right lower lobe.

The right middle lobe bronchus arises from the anterolateral wall of the bronchus intermedius and extends anteriorly and laterally for about 1–2 cm before dividing into medial and lateral segments. The lateral segmental bronchus is visualized over a greater distance, and the medial segment has a more oblique course. Beyond the origin of the superior segment, the right lower lobe divides into anterior, posterior, medial, and lateral segments as seen Figure 4.6 in flexible bronchoscopy and chest CT.

Left Bronchial Tree

The left main bronchus is approximately 4–4.5 cm in length and tends to progress posteriorly, inferiorly, and laterally. It divides into left upper and lower lobe bronchi as seen in Figure 4.7 on flexible bronchoscopy and chest CT. The left main bronchus is much longer than the right and is radiologically seen in three to four contiguous sections below the carina. The upper

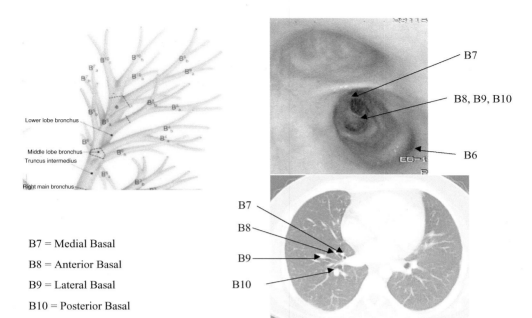

B7 = Medial Basal

B8 = Anterior Basal

B9 = Lateral Basal

B10 = Posterior Basal

Figure 4.6 Right lower lobe.

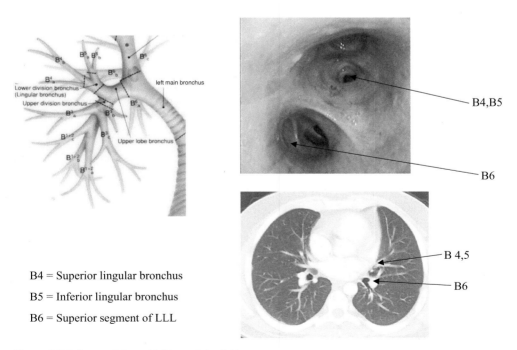

B4 = Superior lingular bronchus

B5 = Inferior lingular bronchus

B6 = Superior segment of LLL

Figure 4.7 Left upper lobe and left lower lobe division.

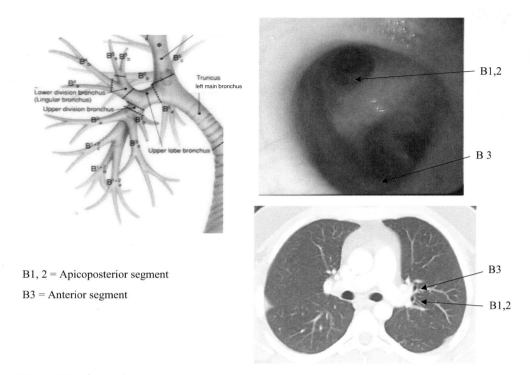

B1, 2 = Apicoposterior segment

B3 = Anterior segment

Figure 4.8 Left upper lobe.

lobe bronchus is 2–3-cm long and divides into upper lobe and lingular divisions. The origin of the left upper lobe bronchus forms a sling over which the left main pulmonary artery passes. The upper lobe division divides into apicoposterior and anterior segmental bronchi as seen in Figure 4.8 on flexible bronchoscopy and chest CT. The anterior segmental bronchus is directed anteriorly and accompanied by the anterior segmental artery. As the upper lobe bronchus extends superiorly, the lingular branch arises and extends slightly downward in an inferolateral direction. The lingular bronchus is about 2–3 cm in length and divides into superior and inferior segmental bronchi.

The superior segment of the left lower lobe bronchus arises immediately on entering into the left lower lobe as seen in Figure 4.7 on flexible bronchoscopy and chest CT. Beyond this, the left lower lobe bronchi is approximately 1 cm in length and divides into anteromedial, lateral, and posterior basilar segments as seen in Figure 4.9 on flexible bronchoscopy and chest CT.

Computed Tomography

Imaging modalities such as multidetector computed tomography (MDCT) complement bronchoscopy and are tools for bronchoscopists to further assess airway anatomy. MDCT can reveal valuable information in planning the bronchoscopy. It can provide detailed analysis of the relationship between the airways, vessels, and mediastinal structures that is useful for bronchoscopy, particularly if a biopsy is planned. Three-dimensional rendering of airways reconstructed from MDCT can also reveal central airway diseases such as tracheal

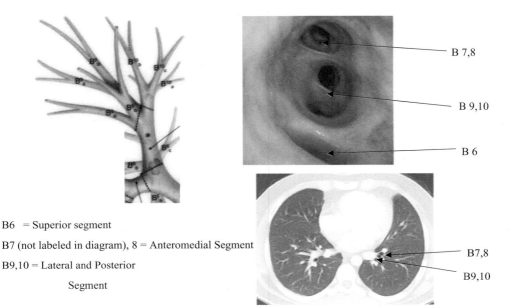

B6 = Superior segment

B7 (not labeled in diagram), 8 = Anteromedial Segment

B9,10 = Lateral and Posterior

       Segment

Figure 4.9 Basilar segment of left lower lobe.

stenosis, congenital tracheal abnormalities, and tracheal and central airway masses. Performing end-inspiratory and dynamic expiratory MDCT can reveal tracheobronchomalacia in the correct clinical context if there is a 50 percent reduction of the airway lumen in cross-section during expiration (see Figures 4.10 and 4.11).

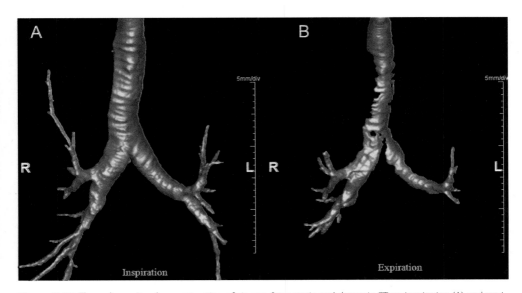

Figure 4.10 Three-dimensional reconstruction of airways from static and dynamic CT on inspiration (A) and expiration (B). Note on expiration the trachea narrows in multiple areas consistent with tracheomalacia.

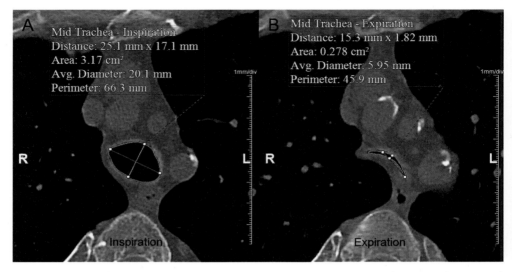

A Mid Trachea - Inspiration
Distance: 25.1 mm x 17.1 mm
Area: 3.17 cm²
Avg. Diameter: 20.1 mm
Perimeter: 66.3 mm

B Mid Trachea - Expiration
Distance: 15.3 mm x 1.82 mm
Area: 0.278 cm²
Avg. Diameter: 5.95 mm
Perimeter: 45.9 mm

Inspiration

Expiration

Figure 4.11 Inspiratory axial CT image reveals patent trachea **(A)**. Dynamic expiratory axial CT **(B)** reveals a narrowed trachea consistent with tracheomalacia.

Conclusion

Solid knowledge of normals and variations in the tracheobronchial anatomy is the key for a successful bronchoscopy. Composite knowledge of adjacent pulmonary vasculature and mediastinal and other structures will aid in performance of specialized diagnostic and therapeutic bronchoscopic procedures.

Further Readings

Boiselle PM. Imaging of the large airways. *Clin Chest Med*. 2008;29(1):181–193.

Lee KS, Boiselle PM. Update on multidetector computed tomography imaging of the airways. *J Thoracic Imaging*. 2010;25(2):112–124.

Letko E. Relapsing polychondritis: a clinical review. *Semin Arthritis Rheum*. 2002;31:384.

Mani SK, Mehta A. Applied anatomy of the airways. In: Wang KP, Mehta AC, Turner JF, eds. *Flexible Bronchoscopy, Part I: Fundamentals of Bronchoscopy*, 2nd ed. Hoboken, NJ: Wiley-Blackwell; 2003; 36–38.

Marks SC, Pasha R. *Rhinology and Paranasal Sinuses, Otolaryngology: Head and Neck Surgery. A Clinical and Reference Guide*, 2nd ed. San Diego: Plural Publishing; 2005.

McDonald TJ. Vasculitis and granulomatous disease. In: McCaffrey TV, ed. *Rhinologic Diagnosis and Treatment*. New York: Thieme; 1996.

Sung A, Williams K, Kovitz K. Endotracheal intubation and tracheostomy. In: Fein AM, Kamholz S, Ost D, eds. *Respiratory Emergencies*. London: Hodder Arnold; 2007;41–56.

Anesthesia for Bronchoscopy

John Pawlowski

Introduction

Instrumentation of the airway is among the most noxious procedures physicians perform. Laryngoscopy and tracheal intubation require 1.3–2.8 times more inhalation anesthesia than does surgical incision. Physiologic responses to bronchoscopy include hypertension, tachycardia, increased cardiac output, laryngospasm, bronchospasm, retching, and vomiting. These hemodynamic and respiratory changes may be well tolerated by healthy individuals, but can lead to myocardial ischemia or respiratory compromise in others. To safely and effectively perform bronchoscopy and other airway procedures, pulmonary specialists must be able to adequately anesthetize the upper airway with local anesthetics, and safely administer moderate (conscious) sedation. This chapter will describe the methods used to anesthetize the oropharynx and upper airway, and the safe use of sedative hypnotics to minimize the frequency and severity of these complications.

Airway Anesthesia

Neuroanatomy of the Airway

Branches of the Vth, IXth, and Xth cranial nerves provide sensation to the airway. The nasal mucosa is innervated by the sphenopalatine plexus, composed of branches of the maxillary branch of the trigeminal nerve. These fibers lie just below the mucosa along the lateral wall of the nares, posterior to the middle turbinate. Sensation to the anterior 2/3 of the tongue is provided by fibers of the mandibular branch of cranial nerve V. The posterior 1/3 of the tongue and the pharyngeal mucosa to the vocal cords are innervated by the glossopharyngeal nerve through the pharyngeal plexus. The superior laryngeal and recurrent laryngeal branches of the vagus innervate the vocal cords, trachea, and bronchi.

Local Anesthetic Techniques

Many of the nerves of the airway can be directly anesthetized by injection or topical application of local anesthetics. Direct injection of the sphenopalatine plexus nerves can be accomplished by injecting 2–3 mL of local anesthetic below the nasal mucosa just posterior to the middle turbinate. However, this technique is impractical and runs the risk of intravascular injection. It also can lead to blood in the airway, obscuring fiber-optic visualization. More commonly, local anesthesia-soaked pledgets or cotton packing is pressed against the mucosa, anesthetizing the underlying nerves. A cotton swab is introduced into the nares and advanced along the turbinate all the way to the posterior wall of the nasal passage. A second swab is then advanced angled slightly more cephalad to the first along the middle turbinate. This swab is more likely to block the sphenopalatine plexus. These pledgets should be kept in place for 2–3 minutes to allow submucosal penetration of the local anesthetic. A 4 percent cocaine solution has traditionally been used for this procedure because of its vasoconstrictive properties, but lidocaine works as well.

The glossopharyngeal nerve can be similarly blocked by either injection or topical administration of local anesthetic at the base of the posterior tonsillar pillar (palatopharyngeal fold). After careful aspiration to prevent injection into the nearby carotid artery, approximately 5 mL of local anesthetic are injected into the submucosa. A 22-gauge, 9-cm needle is used, and the last 1 cm is bent to facilitate injection behind the pillar. Alternatively, cotton pledgets soaked in local anesthetics can be placed at the base of the posterior tonsillar pillar. Care must be taken not to inject too anteriorly, or the hypoglossal nerve can be blocked and motor function of the tongue impaired.

The internal branch of the superior laryngeal nerve can be blocked where it pierces the thyrohyoid membrane, halfway between the hyoid bone and the superior border of the thyroid cartilage. With the patient's neck extended, the hyoid bone is moved laterally. The overlying skin is prepped with an alcohol wipe. A 25-gauge, 2.5-cm needle is advanced until it contacts the superior cornu of the hyoid bone, and is then walked off the cornu inferiorly. It is then advanced another 2–3 mm. As the needle passes through the thyrohyoid membrane, a loss of resistance or "pop" is felt. At that point, approximately 3 mL of local anesthetic are injected deep and superficial to the membrane. Alternatively, the needle can be advanced until air is aspirated and then withdrawn to the submucosal space and the medication injected. The procedure is then repeated on the contralateral side. Care must be taken to avoid intravascular injection into the carotid artery.

Finally, the trachea can be anesthetized by injection of lidocaine through the cricothyroid membrane. With the patient supine, the skin over the membrane is sanitized with an alcohol wipe, and a 22- or 20-gauge needle is used to puncture the membrane. Approximately 4 mL of 2 percent lidocaine is then quickly injected during maximal exhalation. Although this technique is simple and very effective, hemorrhage and even death have been reported because of laceration of small arteries in the cricothyroid membrane.

Although the nerve blocks and injections described earlier are all effective, they require multiple steps and can be unpleasant for the patient. Therefore, techniques that simply deliver the local anesthetics topically to the mucosa of the airway are more common. Several such techniques exist. First, the patient can be asked to gargle and "swish" a 2 percent viscous lidocaine solution. This technique can effectively anesthetize the tongue, mouth, and posterior pharynx. Alternatively, a nebulizer can be used to deliver aerosolized local anesthetic from the mouth to the lungs. Approximately 10 mL of 4 percent lidocaine is administered through a standard nebulizer. This technique is well tolerated, effective as the sole technique in 50 percent of patients, and may be associated with lower plasma levels compared with direct endobronchial administration; however, nebulized lidocaine may not decrease the amount of supplemental lidocaine needed by direct, endobronchial injection, and high serum levels have been described with this technique. Various sprays and atomizers can be used to directly spray the posterior pharynx. After the tongue has been sprayed, it can be grasped with gauze and the spray device inserted into the posterior pharynx. The patient is asked to take deep breaths, and local anesthetic is sprayed during inspiration. Commercially available products can be used to administer benzocaine, or a standard atomizer can be filled with lidocaine for this technique.

Table 5.1 Local Anesthetics

Drug	Maximum Dose	Concerns
Lidocaine	• 4–9 mg/kg (37,40) • 200–400 mg max dose (25,87) • <175 mg/m² (20)	• Seizures • Ventricular tachydysrhythmias • Sedation
Benzocaine	1–2 s spray of Cetacaine or Hurricane (9)	• Methemoglobinemia
Cocaine	1 mg/kg (4)	• Hypertension • Tachycardia • Myocardial ischemia and infarction

Finally, the bronchoscopist can simply use the "spray-as-you-go" method, administering the local anesthetic through the working port of the scope. Lidocaine (4 percent) is used most frequently above the vocal cords with this method, whereas 2 percent lidocaine is generally used below the cords. One report found this technique superior to nebulized lidocaine. All of the techniques described earlier for anesthetizing the airway are effective and safe when properly employed. Comparisons between them have not demonstrated that one is clearly superior to another.

Local Anesthetic Drugs and Their Complications

Several local anesthetics have been described for airway anesthesia, including lidocaine, tetracaine, benzocaine, and cocaine (see Table 5.1). Of these, 2 percent and 4 percent lidocaine are the most common. Irrespective of the technique used for airway anesthesia, the bronchoscopist must be vigilant in watching for signs and symptoms of local anesthetics toxicity. During a nerve block technique, the intra-arterial injection of even a small amount of local anesthetic into the carotid artery can cause seizures and other central nervous system (CNS) toxicity. Topical techniques can lead to the absorption of large quantities of the local anesthetic and to systemic toxicity. The signs and symptoms of local anesthetic toxicity are described in Table 5.2. When doses of 300–400 mg of lidocaine are used, serum lidocaine levels are generally well below toxic levels. The serum concentration is directly related to the dose of local anesthetic administered, and symptoms generally occur when the serum level is >5 mg/L. However, clinicians frequently administer more than the recommended doses without apparent complications, with doses exceeding 600 mg being published. The apparent relative safety of these larger doses is probably due to the fact that 88–92 percent of the drug administered by a nebulizer is wasted. Nonetheless, high serum lidocaine levels, seizures, and even death from local anesthetic toxicity have been described.

The use of benzocaine spray or cocaine solution raises other specific concerns. Benzocaine metabolism in the blood can lead to the formation of methemoglobinemia. Although

Table 5.2 Signs and Symptoms of Local Anesthetic Toxicity

Early Signs and Symptoms	Late Signs and Symptoms
Metallic taste	Somnolence
Tinnitus	Sedation
Anxiety	Seizure
Light-headedness	Ventricular arrhythmia (V. Tach and V. Fib)
	Cardiovascular collapse

this is a relatively rare complication, severe cyanosis, arterial desaturation to levels below 40 percent, and death have been reported. Methemoglobin levels above 30 percent are common. Use of a benzocaine spray (compared with other gel or solution applications) increases the likelihood of methemoglobinemia, and might occur after only a single use. Treatment includes supplemental oxygen and intravenous (IV) methylene blue (1 mg/kg). Cocaine is frequently used for topical anesthesia of the nose. Its effects on the cardiovascular system are well-known. Myocardial ischemia and infarction have been described after topical cocaine administration to the airway.

The administration of anticholinergic agents, such as atropine or glycopyrrolate, is frequently recommended to decrease secretions, improve visibility, and enhance the efficacy of topical local anesthetics. Although this practice is not recommended prior to bronchoscopy, it remains common. Randomized trials have demonstrated that these medications do not improve the quality of airway anesthesia or bronchoscopic view. Higher serum lidocaine concentrations have been reported after the use of atropine. Clinicians should be wary of the potential complications from the tachycardia caused by these medications.

Moderate Sedation

Introduction

Adequate local anesthesia allows the clinician to perform flexible, bronchoscopy without the addition of sedatives or anxiolytics, and the concomitant administration of moderate (conscious) sedation during this procedure is controversial. Conflicting data exist as to whether sedation improves patient tolerance of the procedure. In addition, many of the complications associated with bronchoscopy, and up to half of the life-threatening events can be attributed to the sedation. Others have suggested that sedation should be routine for bronchoscopy. Irrespective of this controversy, a large majority of physicians routinely administer sedation during bronchoscopy. Thus, it is incumbent on the bronchoscopist to understand the regulatory requirements, risks, benefits, medication dosages, monitoring requirements, and impact of patient disease states to safely administer moderate sedation.

Definition and Oversight

Many local, state, and national agencies have published recommendations, guidelines, and standards for the administration of sedation. The clinician must become familiar with these regulations and any local hospital policies regulating the practice of sedation. The American Society of Anesthesiologists (ASA) has published guidelines for the administration of sedation and analgesia by nonanesthesiologists. These guidelines define a continuum of sedation depth, ranging from minimal sedation (anxiolysis) to general anesthesia, as described below.

- **Anxiolysis:** A drug-induced state during which patients respond normally to verbal commands. Although cognitive function and coordination may be impaired, ventilator and cardiovascular functions are unaffected.
- **Moderate sedation/analgesia (previously called conscious sedation):** A drug-induced depression of consciousness during which patients respond purposefully to verbal commands, either alone or accompanied by light tactile stimulation. No interventions are required to maintain a patent airway, and spontaneous ventilation is adequate.

Cardiovascular function is usually maintained (withdrawal from a noxious stimulus is not purposeful movement).
- **Deep sedation:** A drug-induced depression of consciousness during which patients cannot be easily aroused but respond purposefully following repeated painful stimulation. The ability to independently maintain ventilatory function may be impaired. Patients may require assistance in maintaining a patent airway, and spontaneous ventilation may be inadequate. Cardiovascular function is usually maintained (withdrawal from a noxious stimulus is not purposeful movement).
- **General anesthesia:** A drug-induced loss of consciousness during which patients are not awakened, even by painful stimuli.

The ASA guideline outlines recommendations for preprocedure patient evaluation, patient monitoring, equipment availability, training of personnel, drug administration, and the recovery and discharge of patients during moderate or deep sedation. A full review of these guidelines is beyond the scope of this chapter, but the pulmonary physician should be familiar with its contents. In addition, The Joint Commission has adopted many of the recommendations of the ASA guideline and uses the same definitions for moderate and deep sedation. Furthermore, nine Joint Commission standards apply directly to the administration of sedation. All clinicians who administer sedation for interventional pulmonary procedures in the United States must comply with these standards:

- **Moderate or deep sedation is provided by qualified personnel.** This indicates that all personnel who administer sedation must be trained in and have privileges for the safe administration of the sedative medications. In addition, they must be trained to rescue the patient from a deeper than expected level of sedation. Advanced Cardiac Life Support (ACLS) training generally fulfills this requirement.
- **Sedation risks and options are discussed prior to administration.** Clinicians frequently include informed consent for sedation on the form for the procedure.
- **A presedation assessment is performed.** This includes a history and physical examination, evidence that the patient is NPO (*nil per os*, i.e., nothing by mouth) in accordance with guidelines, and specific comorbidities that might impact the safe conduct of the sedation are identified. It also includes a determination that the patient is an appropriate candidate for the procedure and sedation and an immediate preinduction reassessment.
- **Moderate or deep sedation is planned.** Many clinicians create a set of sedation orders that they can complete prior to the procedure.
- **Each patient's physiologic status is monitored during sedation.** See section on monitoring.
- **Each patient's postprocedure status is assessed on admission to and before discharge from the postsedation recovery area.**
- **Patients are discharged from the postsedation recovery area by a licensed, independent practitioner (LIP) or according to criteria approved by the medical staff.** Most institutions create specific, objective criteria for home discharge or to an inpatient unit for patients who receive sedation. These criteria should include an adult escort home and postsedation instructions (including 24-hour contact information). The clinician must be aware that he or she is still responsible for the safe discharge of the patient, even if the patient has been sent home by a nurse in accordance with hospital criteria.

- **Each patient's physiologic status while undergoing moderate or deep sedation is collected and analyzed.** Many institutions have created a form, much like an anesthesia record, for documenting the conduct of moderate or deep sedation.
- **Outcomes of patients undergoing moderate or deep sedation are collected and analyzed.**

Many other organizations, including the American Association of Respiratory Care, the Association of Operating Room Nurses, the American College of Emergency Physicians, and others, have published guidelines and standards regarding sedation to which the pulmonary physician may be held.

Preprocedure Assessment

The ASA moderate sedation guidelines and The Joint Commission standards require that all patients undergoing moderate or deep sedation have a presedation medical assessment. In addition to a standard history and physical examination, this assessment should include information specific to the safe conduct of moderate sedation:

- Evidence that the patient is NPO in accordance with recommended guidelines
- Assessment of the airway (see below)
- Determination of the ASA Physical Status score (see below)
- Evaluation for abnormalities of any major organ system that could negatively impact the safe conduct of sedation
- Determination that the patient has an adult escort home (for those undergoing an outpatient procedure)
- History of adverse experience with sedation
- Consent for sedation (this may be included in the procedural consent)

Assessment of the airway is important because it helps identify those patients in whom endotracheal intubation may be difficult or impossible if they were to become oversedated. The Mallampati classification is one way to identify patients who might be difficult to intubate. To perform this evaluation, ask the patient to open his or her mouth fully and extend the tongue without phonating. The classification is as follows:

- Class I: The entire tonsillar pillars are visible, as is the posterior pharynx
- Class II: The top half of the tonsillar pillars can be seen
- Class III: The tonsillar pillars cannot be seen, but the base of the uvula is visible
- Class IV: Only the hard palate can be seen

Other physical markers of a potentially difficult intubation include a receding mandible, limited mouth opening (<3.5 cm between upper and lower incisors), pronounced overbite of the maxillary incisors, a decreased thyromental distance, and a history of a difficult or failed intubation. Patients deemed to be at significantly increased risk for difficult intubation may benefit from having an anesthesiologist perform the procedural sedation.

The physician who administers moderate or deep sedation must also understand the impact that comorbid diseases may have on the safe conduct of the sedation. Although bronchoscopy with sedation has been performed on patients with significant comorbidities, including obesity, pregnancy, brain lesions, and coronary disease, having such concurrent medical conditions increases the likelihood of complications from the sedation. A full review of the impact of coexisting disease on sedation is beyond the scope of this chapter, but several

Table 5.3 ASA Physical Status

ASA class	Definition	Examples
Class I	No organic, physiologic, biochemical, or physical disturbances. Process for which the procedure is being performed is localized	Healthy patient
Class II	Mild to moderate systemic disturbance caused either by the condition to be treated or other process	Controlled hypertension, mild asthma, AODM, stable (mild) CAD
Class III	Severe systemic disturbance from whatever cause. Impacts daily function	CAD, COPD, compensated CHF, SLE
Class IV	Life-threatening systemic disturbance	Unstable CAD, end-stage renal failure, severe CHF/COPD, long-standing IDDM with end-organ involvement
Class V	Moribund. Not expected to survive 24 h with or without therapy	Ruptured AAA, gunshot wound, severe sepsis

Note: AODM, adult-onset diabetes mellitus; CAD, coronary artery disease; COPD, chronic obstructive pulmonary disease; CHF, congestive heart failure; SLE, systemic lupus erythematosus; IDDM, insulin-dependent diabetes mellitus; AAA, abdominal aortic aneurysm.

points can be made. First, the ASA Physical Status should be determined for each patient receiving moderate or deep sedation (see Table 5.3). Perioperative and anesthesia-related mortality correlates well with increasing ASA class. Many institutions restrict the administration of sedation by nonanesthesiologists to patients who are ASA Class III or below. Furthermore, the Joint Commission may deem this an indication that the patient was assessed and found to be an appropriate candidate for the procedure and sedation. Second, those patients with significant comorbidities should have their disease processes maximally controlled prior to the administration of sedation. When appropriate, a multidisciplinary team approach should be employed, and consultation with an anesthesiologist should be considered. Finally, several disease processes place the patient at significant risk for complications from sedation (see Table 5.4). The pulmonary physician should use extreme caution when administering sedation to these patients.

Equipment and Monitoring

Bronchoscopy and other interventional pulmonary procedures are highly technical and require advanced equipment. In addition, the safe conduct of moderate or deep sedation requires that specific equipment be readily available, irrespective of the degree of complexity of the medical procedure. Table 5.5 describes the recommended equipment needed specifically for sedation.

Although the equipment outlined is important, the vigilance of a clinician monitoring the patient while under sedation is the most important factor influencing patient safety during moderate sedation. Inadequate monitoring of patients has been cited as both too common and a frequent cause of adverse events during bronchoscopy. The monitor, generally a nurse, should have no other significant clinical duties and must have the same training and privileging in the safe administration of sedation and rescue techniques as does the physician performing the procedure. The monitor should continuously evaluate the patient's respiratory rate, cardiac rate and rhythm, blood pressure, oxygen saturation, level of consciousness, and skin condition. These parameters should be documented every

Table 5.4 Risk for Complications from Sedation

Comorbidity	Sedation Risk
Obesity/sleep apnea	• Central sensitivity to sedatives • Rapid arterial desaturation • Difficulty with mask ventilation or intubation
Hypertension	• Increased rate of hypertension • Exaggerated hypotension from vasodilating effect of medications
Systolic cardiac dysfunction	• Slow circulatory time. Delayed effects of sedatives • Prone to pulmonary edema with IV fluids or hemodynamic consequences of bronchoscopy
Ischemic heart disease	• Myocardial ischemia or infarction • Less when supplemental oxygen is used
Aortic valve stenosis	• Limited ability in increase cardiac output in response to hypotension from medications • Increased myocardial oxygen demand from left ventricular hypertrophy. Demand ischemia from hypotension or tachycardia
Dementia	• Increased sensitivity to sedatives • Delayed recovery • Paradoxical agitation is common (reversal agents may help) • Dose slowly and small
Pregnancy	• Aortocaval compression at 20 wk. 15° left uterine displacement • Benzodiazepines were once thought to cause cleft lip/palate. Probably not true. • Uteroplacental circulation and fetal well-being
Chronic pain	• Tolerance. May require very high narcotic dose • Naloxone contraindicated for oversedation

Table 5.5 Recommended Equipment

Category	Specific Equipment
Airway	• Laryngoscopes: Multiple sizes • Endotracheal tubes: Multiple sizes with stylettes • Laryngeal airway mask • Oxygen source and appropriate tubing, masks, or nasal cannulae • Bag/mask ventilation device • Suction with appropriate suction device (Yankauer) • Oral and nasal airways: Multiple sizes
Monitoring	• Noninvasive blood pressure device • Electrocardiograph • Pulse oximeter • Capnograph (required for intubated patients)
Emergency	• Cardiac defibrillator • ACLS medications • Reversal agents (naloxone, flumazenil)
Intravenous access	• Gloves • Tourniquets • Alcohol wipes • IV catheters: Multiple sizes • IV tubing with needleless access ports • Tape • Appropriate IV fluids

Note: Adapted from Godwin SA, Caro DA, Wolf SJ, et al.

5 minutes on a flow sheet designed specifically for moderate sedation (this document can be incorporated into the procedural documentation). In addition, the monitor should document the timing, dose, and indication for all medications administered and the amount of IV fluid administered. Recent literature has suggested the use of expiratory CO_2 monitoring as a way to objectively measure respiration.

Most of the physiologic parameters monitored during sedation are objective and relatively easy to measure. However, both the adequacy of respiration and the level of sedation can be more subjective and prone to error. Simply observing the rise and fall of the chest as a measure of respiration may be misleading as upper airway obstruction caused by oversedation does not prevent chest wall movement. Thus, a patient may have no alveolar ventilation despite apparently normal chest wall movement. Even observing the presence of condensation on the oxygen mask during exhalation does not adequately assess minute ventilation or the presence of oversedation. Furthermore, the use of a full face mask is impractical during bronchoscopy. Given these limitations, the use of expired CO_2 monitors during moderate sedation has been recommended. This monitor identifies hypoventilation and patients at risk for hypoxemia before other clinical markers and with nearly 100 percent sensitivity. In one series, clinicians identified poor ventilation in only 3 percent of cases, whereas CO_2 monitoring found that 56 percent of patients were hypoventilated. More important, active intervention based on early detection of mild hypoventilation as indicated by expiratory CO_2 can effectively prevent subsequent hypoxia. Although measuring true end-tidal CO_2 may be impossible during bronchoscopy in a nonintubated patient, nasal cannula devices with side-port CO_2 detection may be used.

Monitoring the level of consciousness is fraught with subjectivity and inaccuracy. The definition of moderate sedation is that patients should respond to verbal commands, perhaps in conjunction with light touch. Furthermore, their protective reflexes should be intact. This standard is highly subjective, and is made more difficult when the protective airway reflexes are blunted by local anesthetics as is the case in bronchoscopy. Semiobjective scoring systems that monitor the patient's response to reproducible stimuli are often advocated, including the Ramsay score, the Continuum of Depth of Sedation Scale (CDSS), and the Observers Assessment of Alertness/Sedation Scale (OAAS). Each of these is based on a point scale, ranging from alert/anxious to unconscious. More recently, some authors have advocated the use of electroencephalogram(EEG-) based physiologic monitoring to obtain more objective sedation data. This monitoring appears to correlate well with the Ramsay scale, OAAS, and CDSS. More importantly, it may allow clinicians to administer less medication and improve patient cooperation. More work needs to be done in this area before EEG-based monitors become standard sedation monitors.

Monitoring of the patient who has received moderate or deep sedation should continue in the postprocedure recovery area. Vital signs should be continually assessed and documented at regular intervals (generally every 1–30 minutes) while the patient is in the recovery area. Patients who received reversal agents (flumazenil or naloxone) should remain in the recovery area for at least two hours after the reversal is administered. For other patients, no predetermined recovery time should be required, but the patient should demonstrate objective evidence of recovery from the sedative medications prior to discharge to an inpatient unit or to home. Aldrete and Kroulik developed the postanesthesia recovery (PAR) scoring system, similar to the Apgar score for newborns, which helps to determine readiness for discharge. This includes assigning 0–2 points for activity level, respiration, circulation consciousness, and oxygen saturation. (The original scoring system evaluated

Table 5.6 Common Medications Used in Sedation and Adult Dosing Schedules

Drug	Dose	Onset	Duration
Bolus type			
Midazolam	.5–2 mg	2 min	30 min
Fentanyl	25–100 μg	5 min	30 min
Ketorolac	15–30 mg	30 min	4–6 h
Infusion type			
Remifentanil	.1–.3 μg/kg/min	1–2 min	
Propofol	25–100 μg/kg/min	1–2 min	

skin color, but this was modified when pulse oximetry became readily available.) When the patients reach a PAR score of 9 or 10, they are ready for discharge to the inpatient unit. Patients with a PAR score of ten may still demonstrate significant impairment from the sedative medications, and thus a second level of assessment has been added to the PAR score to determine readiness for discharge home. This postanesthesia discharge (PAD) score includes assigning 0–2 points for the dressing, the level of pain, the ability to ambulate, the ability to drink liquids, and urine output. When the sum of the PAR and PAD scores is 18 or greater, the patient is ready for discharge. These scoring systems are used in dozens of countries and are accepted by The Joint Commission.

The medical center should develop specific discharge criteria based on the PAR and PAD score or other objective criteria. Independent licensed practitioners can then discharge patients in accordance with these criteria. Prior to final discharge home, patients and their families should be given verbal and written instructions regarding diet, level of activity and medications, and a 24-hour contact number in case of emergencies. All patients should be discharged in the presence of a responsible adult who will escort them home.

Medications

Introduction

Moderate sedation represents a middle ground between the responsive and cooperative conditions of the lightly sedated patient and the unconscious, anesthetized condition of the patient under general anesthesia. Light sedation can always be augmented by the effective use of topical local anesthesia to numb the oropharynx and blunt the airway reflexes. During optimal situations, moderate sedation allows the patient to be comfortable, sleepy, amnestic, and stable hemodynamically with a modicum of medications. During difficult times, the patient is agitated, semiconscious, uncooperative, and tachycardic. Choosing the anesthetic medications to achieve optimal results requires an understanding of the kinetics and effects of each agent with its potential side effects and the patience to deliver divided doses and to titrate to effect. This section will review some of the commonly used medications in the delivery of moderate sedation to patients who are to undergo airway procedures (See Table 5.6.).

Benzodiazepines

Midazolam is the most appropriate and commonly used benzodiazepine medication for moderate sedation. The combination of amnesia, anxiolysis, and sedation make midazolam an ideal drug either alone or in combination for moderate sedation during procedures that are of short duration and without significant painful stimulation. Midazolam may be administered intravenously orally, intramuscularly, or rectally. Unlike the more lipid-soluble benzodiazepines lorazepam and diazepam, midazolam is not diluted in propylene glycol. This additive is associated with pain on injection and thrombophlebitis. In sedative doses, midazolam reaches peak effect in two minutes and produces sedation for 30 minutes. The rapid onset and short duration make midazolam a useful drug for moderate sedation by bolus injection or infusion.

All benzodiazepines act on the γ-aminobutyric acid (GABA) receptors by enhancing their affinity for GABA. The actions of GABA are to produce both sedation and anxiolysis [73]. Other drugs that act on GABA, such as barbiturates, etomidate, and propofol, can act synergistically to enhance the effects of the benzodiazepines. Other CNS depressants, such as opioids, anesthetic vapors, and α-2 agonists, also have synergistic effects when combined with a benzodiazepine.

Anterograde amnesia is an important component of all benzodiazepines. These agents produce amnestic effects that are out of proportion to the sedative effects. For example, patients may appear alert and conversant, but may remain amnestic for postoperative conversations and instructions. The condition is anterograde (not retrograde) amnesia, and this distinction is frequently misstated. Although the event that is forgotten has occurred in the past, the storage of that event in a patient's memory happens after the administration of midazolam, and thus is properly termed anterograde amnesia. Benzodiazepine cannot reliably cause patients to forget events that occurred before the medication was administered.

Midazolam should be used with caution in elderly patients or in patients with impaired liver function. Midazolam is highly protein bound and is cleared by the liver; therefore, patients with decreased concentrations of serum albumin or with decreased cytochrome P-450 enzymatic activity will have exaggerated effects and duration of activity. Agents that either raise or lower the cytochrome P-450 activity will also affect the action of midazolam. Sedative doses should be administered in a divided fashion, leaving sufficient time to assess the clinical effect of each interval dose. Midazolam does have a reversal agent, flumazenil, which will be discussed later.

Opioids

Although the opioid class of drugs includes dozens of medications with natural and synthetic origins, the major differences consist of their potencies and their rates of equilibration. All opioids are μ-receptor agonists, and this action accounts for their analgesic properties. In addition to the desired analgesic and antitussive effects, all μ-agonists share the side effects of nausea, vomiting, itching, muscle rigidity, and respiratory depression. The use of preemptive antiemetics has been shown to prevent the nausea and vomiting caused by opioids. Fentanyl has been shown to cause chest wall muscular rigidity more often than other synthetic opioids. In some cases, the chest wall rigidity is so severe that it can compromise ventilation and can only be successfully treated with the administration of neuromuscular blocking agents (paralytics). To be effective for moderate sedation, opioids should have high potency and rapidly reach equilibration. Fentanyl and remifentanil possess these properties.

Fentanyl is highly protein bound, lipid soluble, and metabolized by the liver. The time to peak analgesic effect following a single IV bolus is five minutes. The lipid solubility facilitates the movement of fentanyl across the blood–brain barrier. A single dose will last 30 minutes.

Much of the initial bolus is taken up by inactive tissue sites in the lung, fat, and skeletal muscle. As these tissue sites become saturated by either repeated doses or by a continuous infusion, the context-sensitive half-life becomes longer. With continued administration of fentanyl, the half-life approaches the elimination half-life of 3–4 hours. Therefore, the advantage of fentanyl as a short-acting agent is lessened as the duration of the procedure requires multiple repeated boluses or a continuous infusion. Specific opioid antagonists do exist and will be discussed later.

An alternative opioid to fentanyl that can be used for both brief procedures and those with varying duration is remifentanil. This opioid is used for general anesthesia only, as remifentanil will cause apnea. Remifentanil is a synthetic opioid with equivalent potency to fentanyl; both are about 100 times more potent than morphine. A rapid onset of analgesic effect occurs after an IV bolus of remifentanil, with peak effect within 1–1.5 minutes. Unlike the other synthetic opioids, remifentanil has a unique degradation, being metabolized by plasma esterases. The elimination half-life is 8–20 minutes and is independent of liver or kidney function. Repeated dosing or continuous infusions do not prolong the elimination half-life. For example, a 5-hour infusion of remifentanil produced return of breathing within 3–5 minutes following discontinuation. Rapid elimination of remifentanil means that it does not provide any residual analgesia in the postoperative period. Other analgesics need to be started in the recovery area.

It is important to realize that all opioids have the unique property of providing intense pain relief without loss of proprioception or consciousness. Although this property has brought comfort to millions, it also brings the possibility of awareness. Intraoperative awareness under general anesthesia is a recognized complication and one that is more common when opioids are used. Awareness during moderate sedation should be an expected condition, but often patients will complain of hearing and feeling portions of their procedure. It is essential that anyone who is planning to administer moderate sedation advise the patient that some degree of recall is to be expected.

Propofol

Under the general heading of sedatives/hypnotics, propofol emerges as a versatile and effective agent to use when administering moderate sedation. Currently the most commonly used parenteral anesthetic agent in the United States, propofol is a substituted isopropylphenol that is insoluble in water and usually prepared in a lipid vehicle for IV administration. The emulsion consists of soybean oil, egg lecithin, and glycerol. Disodium ethylene diamine tetraacetic acid (EDTA) or sodium metabisulfite is added as a preservative and to inhibit bacterial growth, but the propofol mixture does support bacterial proliferation and serious infections have been reported.

As with the benzodiazepines and other sedatives/hypnotics, propofol acts on the GABA receptors and decreases the dissociation rate of GABA from the receptor. Metabolized in the liver by cytochrome P-450, there is also extensive nonhepatic metabolism as well as inactive tissue uptake. As a result of these elimination pathways, the context-sensitive half-life is not prolonged in such conditions as a propofol infusion lasting 8 hours. Propofol concentrations are not elevated in cirrhotic or alcoholic patients (suggesting the ability of the extrahepatic pathways to metabolize propofol) nor in patients with renal failure, but concentrations are higher in elderly patients.

Propofol produces rapid sedation without associated nausea or vomiting and a rapid return of cognitive function. Either an infusion or incremental boluses every five minutes can create levels of moderate sedation. The potential side effects of propofol include hypotension, apnea, and airway obstruction, so the patient needs to have close hemodynamic monitoring and immediate access to emergency airway interventions. Propofol does not seem to provoke bronchospasm. It often produces pain at the injection site, but this pain incidence can be reduced to <10 percent with the administration into a large vein (e.g., antecubital) or pretreatment with 1 percent lidocaine or opioids. The use of propofol by health care providers other than anesthetists is controversial. Many states require that the providers be certified in sedation techniques and competent in managing the airway.

Severe lactic acidosis as a consequence of prolonged propofol administration has been described in both adults and children. Although initially described with propofol infusions lasting more than 24 hours, there have been a number of reports of acidosis developing in shorter durations. Any patient on a propofol infusion with an unexplained tachycardia should be suspected of having "propofol infusion syndrome." The arterial blood gas and serum lactate levels should indicate a metabolic acidosis. Other causes of metabolic acidosis – such as tourniquet release, diabetic ketoacidosis, sepsis, and hyperchloremic metabolic acidosis from extensive infusions of normal saline – should be excluded. Treatment includes discontinuation of the propofol and supportive care, which has included extracorporeal membrane oxygenation in at least one report. The mechanism for propofol infusion syndrome appears to be interruption of the electron transport chain and impairment of the long-chain fatty acid metabolism.

Nonsteroidal Antiinflammatory Drugs (NSAIDs)

The NSAIDs share the three properties of acting as analgesics, antiinflammatories, and antipyretics. Although a larger, heterogeneous group of medications exists in this category, ketorolac is the only applicable drug to the administration of moderate sedation. As one of the few NSAIDs approved for parenteral use, ketorolac has greater analgesic activity than antiinflammatory activity. As a traditional NSAID, ketorolac does block cyclooxygenase-1 and therefore does promote gastric ulceration and platelet inhibition.

Administered as a sole analgesic or in combination with opioids to potentiate the analgesic effect, ketorolac provides rapid pain relief. Ketorolac does not induce tolerance nor does it cause respiratory depression. In patients with an aspirin allergy, nasal polyposis, or asthma, ketorolac has been reported to trigger life-threatening bronchospasm. Patients with congestive heart failure, hypovolemia, or hepatorenal syndrome may be susceptible to ketorolac-induced renal failure because of their dependence on local renal prostaglandin production to maintain renal blood flow.

Antiemetics

The sensation of nausea and act of emesis are a coordinated set of muscular, autonomic, behavioral, and emotional responses that exist to rid the stomach of toxins. In clinical practice, nausea and vomiting are unpleasant and unintended consequences to anesthesia, inflammation, or motion that can add morbidity to and complicate the recovery from any procedure. The coordination of the vomiting response occurs in the central emesis center in the lateral reticular formation of the mid brainstem in the area adjacent to both the chemoreceptor trigger zone (CTZ), found in the area postrema at the base of the fourth ventricle, and the nucleus solitarius of the vagal nerve. The CTZ monitors the cerebrospinal fluid for toxins and receives information from the gut. The emesis center also receives information from the cerebral cortex regarding anticipatory nausea and vestibular input with respect to motion sickness.

This complex neural connection has a variety of neurotransmitter influences. Serotonin, histamine, acetylcholine, dopamine, and prostaglandins have key roles in the neural modulation of the emesis center. The antiemetic strategy, therefore, can be targeted at one or several of these neural modulators. For example, ondansetron can block the specific 5-hydroxytryptamine-3 receptors in the CTZ, and the antihistamine cyclizine or the antimuscarinic scopolamine can block the vestibular input from motion sickness. A steroid such as dexamethasone can block the emetogenic influence from inflammation, and benzodiazepines can suppress anticipatory nausea. Therefore, the cause of the nausea may differ in different patients, and the effective treatment may address the particular etiology. Often, however, multiple medications that use a variety of mechanisms of action are required to reduce the symptoms of nausea and prevent vomiting.

Ondansetron is structurally similar to serotonin, and an IV dose reaches peak effect within 30–60 minutes. Interestingly, the drug conveys antiemetic action long after it has disappeared from the plasma circulation, suggesting a continued interaction at the serotonin receptor. For this reason, all the serotonin antagonists may be given once daily. Metabolized in the liver by cytochrome P-450 enzymes, ondansetron should be reduced in patients with liver failure, although no such reduction is needed in elderly patients. Ondansetron is effective for nausea from chemotherapy and postoperative sources but is ineffective in treating motion sickness. Side effects from ondansetron are usually headache and diarrhea. The usual dose of ondansetron in the postoperative setting is 4 mg IV. Higher doses do not show greater reduction of postoperative nausea and vomiting.

Reversal Agents

All medication antagonists have their own chemical properties, kinetics, binding characteristics, and elimination pathways. The constellation of characteristics will determine how well the antagonist can reverse the action of the agonist, but also will determine what other concerns the practitioner should have in the process of using a reversal agent.

An imidazolebenzodiazepine, flumazenil binds with high affinity to sites on the GABA-A receptor. Flumazenil, when combined with a benzodiazepine, does not produce water. In other words, all drugs have side effects, and using one to reverse the effects of another does not come without some risk. Flumazenil competitively inhibits the binding of both agonists and reverse agonists to the GABA-A receptor. Slight activity, which resembles a reverse agonist at low concentrations and an agonist at high concentrations, has been reported. The agonist activity of flumazenil, however, does not prevent the withdrawal symptoms that have been reported. Just as withdrawal from chronic benzodiazepine use can cause a variety of effects, flumazenil can cause dysphoria, irritability, anorexia, sweating tremors, unpleasant dreams, dizziness, exacerbation of insomnia or anxiety, and frank seizures. Flumazenil is not recommended in patients who are taking antiseizure medication.

Usually, 1–5 mg of flumazenil is given in divided doses between one and ten minutes until the desired reversal of sedation is achieved. The clinical effects last from 30 to 60 minutes and, therefore, the potential for resedation is possible and the flumazenil may need to be rebolused or an infusion started. If 5 mg of flumazenil does not reverse sedation, the sedation was probably not caused by benzodiazepine overdose. In practice, benzodiazepine overdose rarely causes respiratory depression, and, therefore, the urgent need for reversal using flumazenil is exceedingly uncommon.

As with flumazenil, the administration of naloxone to reverse the effects of opioids does not produce water. A nonselective competitive antagonist, naloxone binds with high affinity to all three opioid receptors (μ, δ, κ). Used to treat narcotic-induced depression of ventilation, the side effect of naloxone is to also reverse narcotic-induced analgesia. Postsurgical patients can develop hyperacute, severe pain. The activation of the sympathetic nervous system in response to naloxone-induced pain can include tachycardia, hypertension, pulmonary edema, and cardiac arrhythmias, including ventricular fibrillation. Plasma cortisol and catecholamine levels rise following naloxone administration. Less obvious side effects from naloxone are decreased performance on memory tests and dysphoria.

Given in divided doses of 1–4 μg/kg, naloxone quickly reverses opioid-induced respiratory depression and has a short duration of action (30–45 minutes). Thus, the effects of naloxone may be shorter than the half-life of the opioid that is causing the respiratory depression. A continuous infusion of naloxone may be necessary and is usually started at 5 (μg/kg)/h.

In clinical practice, careful titration of the opioid medications with understanding of the time to peak activity and the potential for respiratory depression should make the use of opioid antagonists uncommon. Opioid doses should be adjusted in elderly patients and in patients with limited hepatic function or poor pulmonary reserve. Opioid doses should be adjusted downward whenever other sedative agents are used in combination. Finally, the narcotic effect should be reserved with naloxone as a rescue strategy when respiratory depression occurs and when mechanical or supplemental breathing measures are not practical or beneficial in improving the situation.

Complications of Sedation

Complications from moderate sedation can occur, from undersedation, oversedation, and idiosyncratic responses to "therapeutic levels" of sedation. Too little sedation can lead to excessive movement, delirium, and pain. Too much sedation can produce hemodynamic collapse and respiratory depression. Even those patients receiving "optimal" therapeutic concentrations of sedation can demonstrate allergic reactions, rigidity, or laryngospasm. Even therapeutic levels of sedatives can worsen such conditions as acute intermittent porphyria, malignant hyperthermia, or carcinoid crisis. Specific complications can occur with specific pharmacologic agents, such as adrenal suppression from etomidate and rhabdomyolysis from propofol. This section will focus on the general complications that occur from oversedation.

Most sedatives are myocardial depressants and/or vasodilators that can act to profoundly lower blood pressure. The degree of cardiovascular depression will depend on the patient's cardiovascular and volume status, any medications that have additive effects on the blood pressure, and any surgical conditions that may affect the patient. For example, the reverse Trendelenburg position can lower the preload and cause an exaggerated hypotensive response to sedatives. Effects on the blood pressure from sedation can be greater in patients with cardiomyopathy, valvular heart disease, or pericardial conditions, such as acute tamponade. Resuscitative drugs should always be immediately available to administer when a sedative is given.

Many sedatives are respiratory depressants and, in large enough doses, can cause apnea. Most sedatives blunt the ventilatory response to both high levels of carbon dioxide and low levels of oxygen. For this reason, all patients who receive sedation need to be monitored for both ventilation and oxygenation. Respiratory rates can be misleading, however, as they may not reflect minute ventilation. For this reason, either minute ventilation or end-tidal CO_2 should be used for deeper sedation techniques, to better detect hypoventilation. For oxygenation status, the pulse oximeter provides a reliable and sensitive predictor of desaturation in most settings. Evidence of hypoxemia may not occur until the patient has been hypoventilating or apneic for several minutes. To rescue patients from conditions of hypoventilation or hypoxemia, advanced airway equipment needs to be immediately available, along with a source of enriched oxygen, continuous suction, and the trained personnel to use them.

In conclusion, the use of moderate sedation to allow the accomplishment of airway procedures requires a balance of anesthetic drugs with their relaxant, sedative, and analgesic effects with the unwanted and potentially dangerous side effects. The conduct of the anesthetic and the recognition of these side effects require planning and monitoring. Every patient needs a history and physical examination, including an examination of the airway. All patients need standard monitoring and a person designated as the monitor. Each bronchoscopic procedure requires the proper equipment, medications, and training to administer the medications and to deal with side effects. Finally, all patients need a safe environment in which to recover from sedation. With careful preparation, proper supplies, and protocols, bronchoscopy can be performed under excellent surgical conditions and with minimal adverse events.

Further Readings

Abdelmalak BB, Gildea TR, Doyle DJ. Anesthesia for bronchoscopy. *Curr Pharm Des*. 2012;18(38): 6314–6324.

Aldrete JA. Post-anesthetic recovery score. *J Am Coll Surg*. 2007;205:e3–e4.

Aldrete JA, Kroulik D. A postanesthetic recovery score. *Anesth Analg*. 1970;49:924–934.

Bahhady IJ, Ernst A. Risks of and recommendations for flexible bronchoscopy in pregnancy: a review. *Chest*. 2004;126:1974–1981.

Burton JH, Harrah JD, Germann CA, Dillon DC. Does end-tidal carbon dioxide monitoring detect respiratory events prior to current sedation monitoring practices? *Acad Emerg Med*. 2006;13: 500–504.

Chisholm CJ, Zurica J, Mironov D, et al. Comparison of electrophysiologic monitors with clinical assessment of level of sedation. *Mayo Clin Proc*. 2006;81:46–52.

Day RO, Chalmers DRC, Williams KM, Campbell TJ. Death of a healthy volunteer in a human research project: implications for Australian clinical research. *Med J Aust*. 1998;168:449–451.

Doenicke AW, Roizen MF, Rau J, et al. Pharmacokinetics and pharmacodynamics of propofol in a new solvent. *Anesth Analg*. 1997;85:1399–1403.

Du Rand IA, Blaikley J, Booton R, Chaudhuri N, Gupta V, Khalid S, Mandal S, Martin J, Mills J, Navani N, Rahman NM, Wrightson JM, Munavvar M. British Thoracic Society guideline for diagnostic flexible bronchoscopy in adults. *Thorax*. 2013;68:i1–i44.

Fudickar A, Bein B, Tonner PH. Propofol infusion syndrome in anaesthesia and intensive care medicine. *Curr Opin Anaesthesiol*. 2006;19:404–410.

Godwin SA, Caro DA, Wolf SJ, et al. Clinical policy: procedural sedation and analgesia in the emergency department. *Ann Emerg Med*. 2005;45:177–196.

Hatton MQF, Allen MB, Vathenen AS, et al. Does sedation help in fiberoptic bronchoscopy? *BMJ*. 1994;309:1206–1207.

Honeybourne D, Neumann CS. An audit of bronchoscopy practice in the United Kingdom: a survey of adherence to national guidelines. *Thorax*. 1997;52:709–713.

Hwang JCF, Hanowell LH, Mott JM, et al. Perioperative bronchoscopy. In: Hanowell LH, Waldron RJ, eds. *Airway Management*. Philadelphia: Lippincott-Raven; 1996.

Isaac PA, Barry JE, Vaughan RS, et al. A jet nebulizer for delivery of topical anesthesia to the respiratory tract: a comparison with cricothyroid puncture and direct spraying for fiberoptic bronchoscopy. *Anaesthesia*. 1990;45:46–48.

The Joint Commission. Pre-induction assessment for sedation and analgesia. Available at: www .jointcommission.org/AccreditationPrograms/Hospitals/Standards/FAQs/Provision+of+Care/ Assessment/Pre_Induction.htm. Accessed November 29, 2007.

Jones DA, McBurney A, Stanley PJ, et al. Plasma concentrations of lignocaine and its metabolites during fiberoptic bronchoscopy. *Br J Anaesth*. 1982;54:853–857.

Jose RJ, Shaefi S, Navani N. Sedation for flexible bronchoscopy: current and emerging evidence. *Eur Respir Rev*. 2013;22(128):106–116.

Anesthesia for bronchoscopy. *Curr Opin Anaesthesiol*. 2014 epub.

Kane GC, Hoehn SM, Behrenbeck TR, Mulvagh SL. Benzocaine-induced methemoglobinemia based on the Mayo Clinic experience from 28,478 transesophageal echocardiograms: incidence, outcomes, and predisposing factors. *Arch Intern Med*. 2007;167:1977–1982.

Kimura T, Watanabe S, Asakura N, et al. Determination of end-tidal sevoflurane concentration for tracheal intubation and minimum alveolar anesthetic concentration in adults. *Anesth Analg*. 1994;79:3780–3781.

Lundgren R, Haggmark S, Reiz S. Hemodynamic effects of flexible fiberoptic bronchoscopy performed under topical anesthesia. *Chest*. 1982;82:295–299.

Matot I, Kramer MR. Sedation in outpatient bronchoscopy. *Respir Med*. 2000;94:1145–1153.

Matot I, Kramer MR, Glantz L, et al. Myocardial ischemia in sedated patients undergoing fiberoptic bronchoscopy. *Chest*. 1997;112:1454–1458.

Makaryus JN, Makaryus AN, Johnson M. Acute myocardial infarction following the use of intranasal anesthetic cocaine. *South Med J*. 2006;99:759–61.

Middleton RM, Shah A, Kirkpatrick MB. Topical nasal anesthesia for flexible bronchoscopy. A comparison of four methods in normal subjects and in patients undergoing transnasal bronchoscopy. *Chest*. 1991;99:1093–1096.

Mulroy MF. Peripheral nerve blockade. In: Barash PG, Cullen BF, Stoelting RK, eds. *Clinical Anesthesia*, 2nd ed. Philadelphia: Lippincott Williams & Wilkins; 1992.

Osula S, Stockton P, Adbelaziz MM, Walshaw MJ. Intratracheal cocaine induced myocardial infarction: an unusual complication of fiberoptic bronchoscopy. *Thorax*. 2003;58:733–734.

Parker MRJ, Day CJE, Coote AH. Sedation in fiberoptic bronchoscopy. *BMJ*. 1995;310:872.

Pathak V, Welsby I, Mahmood K, Wahidi M, MacIntyre N, Shofer S. Ventilation and anesthetic approaches for rigid bronchoscopy. *Ann Am Thorac Soc*. 2014;11(4):628–634.

Puruggganan RV. Intravenous anesthesia for thoracic procedures. *Curr Opin Anaesthesiol*. 2008; 21(1): 1–7.

Ramsay MAE, Savege TM, Simpson BRI, Goodwin R. Controlled sedation with alphaxolone-alphadolone. *BMJ*. 1974;ii:656–658.

Reed AP. Preparation of the patient for awake flexible fiberoptic bronchoscopy. *Chest*. 1992;101: 244–253.

Riker RR, Picard JT, Fraser GL. Prospective evaluation of the Sedation-Agitation Score for adult critically ill patients. *Crit Care Med.* 1999;27:1325–1329.

Ross AF, Ferguson JS. Advances in interventional pulmonology. *Curr Opin Anaesthesiol.* 2009;22(1): 11–17.

Sarkiss M. Anesthesia for bronchoscopy and interventional pulmonology: from moderate sedation to jet ventilation. *Curr Opin Pulm Med.* 2011;17(4):274–278.

Schreiber F. Austrian Society of Gastroenterology and Hepatology–guideline on sedation and monitoring during gastrointestinal endoscopy. *Endoscopy.* 2007;39:259–262.

Simpson FG, Arnold AG, Purvis A, et al. Postal survey of bronchoscopy practice by physicians in the United Kingdom. *Thorax.* 1986;411:311–317.

Smith CM, Stead RJ. Survey of flexible fiberoptic bronchoscopy in the United Kingdom. *Eur Respir J.* 2002;19:458–463.

Stoelting K, Hillier S, eds. *Pharmacology & Physiology in Anesthetic Practice.* Philadelphia: Lippincott Williams & Wilkins; 2006.

Stolz D, Chhajed PN, Leuppi J, et al. Nebulized lidocaine for flexible bronchoscopy: a randomized, doubleblind, placebo-controlled trial. *Chest.* 2005;128:1756–1760.

Villegas T. Sleep apnea and moderate sedation. *Gastroenterol Nurs.* 2004;27:121–124.

Wahidi M, Jain P, Jantz M, et al. ACCP consesnsus statement on the use of topical anesthesia, analgesia, and sedation during flexible bronchoscopy in adult patients. *Chest.* 2011;140:1342–1350.

Weaver CS, Hauter WH, Duncan CE, et al. An assessment of the association of bispectral index with 2 clinical sedation scales for monitoring depth of procedural sedation. *Am J Emerg Med.* 2007;25: 918–924.

Williams KA, Barker GL, Harwood RJ, Woodall NM. Combined nebulization and spray-as-you-go topical local anaesthesia of the airway. *Br J Anaesth.* 2005;95:549–553.

Wolf A, Weir P, Setage P, et al. Impaired fatty acid oxidation in propofol infusion syndrome. *Lancet.* 2001;357:606–607.

Chapter 6

Anatomy and Care of the Bronchoscope

Robert Garland

The flexible bronchoscope has undergone many technological advances since it was first introduced almost 50 years ago. Despite these advances in imaging and ease of use, it remains a fragile piece of equipment and susceptible to damage. If improvements can be made to the quality of the image and the size of the working channel without compromising the overall diameter of the instrument, why can't significant improvements be made to the durability of the bronchoscope? Simply put, there is so much technology stuffed into such a small compartment that even slight trauma to the instrument can be devastating.

It is truly remarkable that this equipment can perform all the functions that it does considering the difficulties in engineering such a small-diameter instrument. Let's review the challenges in developing the flexible bronchoscopes that are available today.

Basic Requirements of the Bronchoscope

The bronchoscope must accomplish several feats with some challenging obstacles that it must overcome:

- It must be small enough to fit into the airway and still provide space for breathing.
- The airway does not have any illumination, so we must provide artificial light to see where we are going.
- There are bifurcations in the airway, so we need a mechanism for steering the instrument.
- The airway can be obstructed with fluid or blood, so we must have a way to clear those to see properly.
- We need a way to take samples of the airway should we see something abnormal.
- It would be helpful to record a finding to share with others by capturing an image of it.

Anatomy and Physiology of the Bronchoscope

Now that we have identified the needs of the bronchoscope, let's take a look at how the current bronchoscopes accomplish this. I would like to distinguish between the anatomy (structure) and the physiology (function) of the instrument (Figure 6.1).

Anatomy

The bronchoscope is designed to be held in the left hand because the universal cord (the part of the scope that plugs into the light source) comes off the left side of the control section of the scope, and the weight of the scope is supported by this hand. There are three basic components to the flexible bronchoscope [3]:

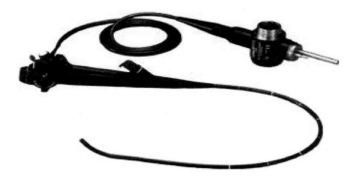

Figure 6.1 Flexible bronchoscope.

- Control section
- Insertion tube
- Universal cord

Control Section

This is the part of the bronchoscope that you hold with your left hand. It is designed so that the operator can perform multiple functions with this hand while still gripping the scope. The right hand should only be used to hold the insertion tube at the area closest to where it enters the patient.

There is a lever that can be moved up or down by the thumb that controls the angle of the distal tip for steering and a valve that can be compressed by the first finger to control the vacuum applied to the airways. Most scopes available today have a separate valve on the control section that allows for placement of accessories for sampling the airway.

Also on the control section is a series of remote switches that can be programmed for a variety of functions such as capturing images, magnifying the field, and even applying different wavelengths of light to the airways.

Insertion Tube

This is the section of the instrument that actually enters the patient and consists of a flexible catheter, which in the adult bronchoscope is between 55 and 60 mm long and usually has an outer diameter of between 4 and 6 mm. Depending on the size of the outer diameter, there is a plastic catheter between 2 and 3 mm traveling through the middle of the insertion tube that is used for passing accessories or sampling fluid or tissue. This is known as the working channel.

Running alongside the catheter are two fiber-optic bundles that carry light from an external light source to provide illumination to the airways where no natural light can reach. There are two thin wires that are connected to a lever in the control body, pass through the insertion tube, and connect at the distal end of the scope to a series of hinged devices that are used for steering the instrument. Whether the scope's imaging system is considered fiber-optic or video chip technology, there are either fiber bundles or several electrical wires that transmit an electronic image through this insertion tube after receiving the image from a small lens at the distal end of the scope. All of these delicate catheters, fibers, cables, and wires are wrapped with a flexible but strong metal sheath to protect them somewhat from the potential damage

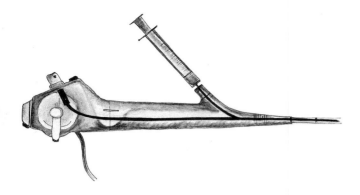

Figure 6.2 Plumbing system.

of human teeth and user error. Outside of this sheath a thin, waterproof membrane is applied to separate the devastating effects of moisture from the internal components.

Universal Cord

This section of the bronchoscope carries information and light to and from the control body, the video processor, and the light source. At one end is a connector that attaches to the external light source and video processor, and the other end provides a support for the hand that holds the instrument as it is permanently connected to the control body.

Physiology

The primary function of the bronchoscope is to provide an inspection of the airways. To accomplish this, many components of the equipment need to work together. The scope functions as a series of independent systems that rely on one another for the smooth operation of the instrument. There are four systems that make up the bronchoscope as we know it today.

Plumbing System

The working channel acts as a conduit for passing accessory instruments for sampling the airways and also as a channel to remove secretions and blood to allow proper viewing. In most bronchoscopes there are two ways to access the working channel. At the top of the control section there is a valve that, when compressed, allows communication between the working channel and a vacuum source that has been attached to the valve. This then applies suction to the channel and clears whatever fluid is in front of the scope. There is usually a second valve on the control section where accessory devices or fluid can be placed through to allow sampling of the lung. This valve works by having a narrow opening in the housing that will close when nothing is in it and will open only enough for the device to pass through. This allows the operator to apply suction even though the channel is partially obstructed with the device. These valves snap on to a seat in the control section and are usually considered single-use items as they are difficult to properly clean (Figure 6.2).

Mechanical System

A series of levers, wires, and hinged metal bands make up the parts of the mechanical system that allow the operator to "steer" his or her instrument to specific locations in the airways.

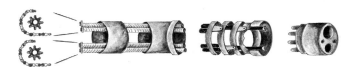

Figure 6.3 Mechanical system.

As described earlier, there is a lever on the control section that can be moved up or down by the thumb that in turn pulls or pushes thin wires running through the insertion tube to the bending section of the scope at the distal tip, which moves this hinged section anterior or posterior relative to the orientation of the scope. This system is similar to the "chain and sprocket system" used to move bicycles. The amount of "angulation" varies depending on the scope but is usually around 180° up and 130° down. Over time, the wires can become stretched and the angulation will become less, and adjustments will need to be made to bring it back to specifications (Figure 6.3).

Electrical System

This system serves many functions in the modern bronchoscope that most of us take for granted. In the video bronchoscope that is commonly used today, the electrical system helps to carry the signals from the video chip to the video processor to be converted to an image that we then understand. It also allows the operator with a press of his or her finger to perform functions on the remote switches like capturing images, magnifying the image, or altering the light to which the tissue is exposed.

One of the most important features is that it provides the feedback from the processor to allow for corrections in areas like light intensity. There is a difference in the light needed to illuminate the airway depending on how close the end of the lens is to the tissue and whether there are secretions in the field reflecting the light. This feedback will reduce the amount of light if the area under inspection is very close to the tissue or if there is excessive reflection from fluid or secretions (Figure 6.4).

Image System

The quality of imaging is truly amazing in the instruments that are in use today, especially when you stop to consider that you may be seeing images on a video monitor with the clarity of high definition taken from a lens that is only a little more than 1 mm wide. To be able to

Figure 6.4 Electrical system.

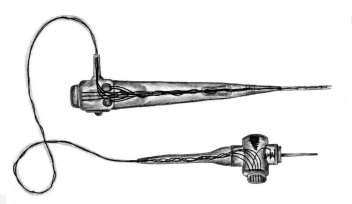

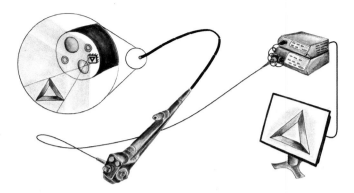

Figure 6.5 Imaging system with monitor.

see deep into a body cavity with this clarity poses many challenges. First, we must provide enough light through a tube that has to be small enough to pass through the adult vocal cords; this requires that the whole tube cannot be much more than 6 mm in diameter. Then we must remember that some of the passages turn back on themselves, so the scope must be able to bend completely 180° without kinking and damaging its components (Figure 6.5).

The airway is illuminated by an external light source that is attached to the bronchoscope. The light is carried through the scope via a series of glass fibers wrapped tightly in a bundle that allows the light to bend around corners. There are two fiber bundles needed to provide enough light to the distal end of the scope so that the light is distributed evenly without it looking like one is shining a flashlight down the airway. This prevents a bright spot in the middle of the field while the edges are progressively dimmer. If one of these fiber bundles is damaged, then you may see an area of brighter concentration of light in one part of the airway.

The very end of the bronchoscope contains a tiny lens that magnifies and focuses the image either on the fiber bundle in a fiber-optic scope or on a video chip in a video system. In the fiber-optic scope, the image is carried through this fiber bundle to another lens that magnifies and refocuses it. In the later video systems, the image is disassembled into light levels and colors and sent back, where it is reassembled into an image in the video processor.

Given that we are viewing this image from a lens that is 1 mm wide, it is remarkable that we have a field of view of 120°. Most of the scopes today have the ability to view the image at a depth of between 3 and 100 mm, so this allows the operator to be very close to the object in question, and is necessary when working in an airway that is only 10–20 mm wide. It is also important to remember that, as we view the image on a monitor, any accessories passed through it will appear at 3 o'clock from the center of the image (Figure 6.5).

Types of Bronchoscopes Available

There are three categories of bronchoscopes which are based on how we visualize the airway.

1. Non-video

These original bronchoscopes transmitted light and images through a series of glass fibers called fiber-optic bundles. This technology allowed a flexible bronchoscopyfor the first time, as prior to this development there was no way to allow light to "bend" as is required with the flexible bronchoscope. The scope had a lens at either end of the fibers to focus and view the airway through an eyepiece. Further developments allowed a video convertor to be attached from the eyepiece to a video processor to visualize the airway on a monitor screen, but the images were inferior to what is available with true video. There are still a small amount of scopes made this way today. Most of them are small-diameter scopes that do not have the physical space in them to allow for video technology.

2. Video

The video bronchoscope was a significant improvement in endoscopic technology by providing better imaging with the use of the charge-coupled device (CCD) chip. This chip, placed directly behind the distal lens, eliminates the fiber-optic bundle. Even though it has the advantage of allowing light to bend, the fiber-optic bundle was no comparison to the CCD chip in the way images can be transmitted. The chip converts the image into electronic signals that are carried via wires to the video processor for reassembly into an image that can be understood by the human eye.

There were many other developments that occurred because of the integration of the bronchoscope and the video processor (white balance, zoom). These developments will be discussed later in this chapter.

3. Hybrid

Because of space limitations, some of the bronchoscopes available in the market today are a combination of the materials that make up the video and non-video instruments. An example would be a small-diameter bronchoscope, the size of which may be necessary for navigating in distal airways and which has superior imaging that would not be available with the non-video scope. The insertion tube (because of its narrow diameter requirements) may not be able to "accept" the size of a CCD chip, so the older fiber-optic bundle may have to be used to transmit imaging through the insertion tube to a point in the control section where a CCD chip could be placed to perform the function of transmitting image technology via an electronic signal to the video processor. The advantage is improved imaging over a true fiber-optic system.

Advances in Scope Technology

Although the bronchoscope may not appear very different over the past several yearsthere have been many improvements that allow for better visualization, navigation, ease of operator use, and improved safety for patients. The latest generation of bronchoscopes are far more versatile than in the past.

Imaging

The imaging systems of today's bronchoscopes are far superior than the original video technology when CCD chips were first used in them. Problems associated with visualizing an image in an environment of artificial light (creating glare and shadows) have been addressed with improvements in feedback mechanisms for better control of brightness and colors. Some scope versions also offer magnification of the tissue image as well as a variety of light exposures for early detection of abnormal tissue surfaces.

But the biggest improvement in imaging design has to be the incorporation of high definition technology into the instrument. Most of the scopes produced today are available in high definition resolution. This crisper, clearer image quality is far superior to those produced in

Table 6.1 Benefits and Limitations Based on Scope Size

Scope Size	Advantages	Limitations
Small	Better Maneuverability	Smaller Channel Size, Inferior Imaging
Large	Larger Working Channel Better Imaging	Inability to Navigate to Distal Airways

the past. You must remember though that purchasing a high definition bronchoscope does not guarantee this imaging without the associated processor, cabling, and monitors.

Navigation

Bronchoscope manufacturing has come a long way in providing bronchoscopes today to meet the needs of most clinical applications. We now have instruments of almost every diameter that will pass into adults and children, with working channels to go along with them that will accept the variety of accessories that are produced for diagnostic and therapeutic procedures. Below is a table (Table 6.1) of the advantages and limitations of using a small vs. a larger diameter scope.

It is important to remember that there are compromises that are made when selecting options for a bronchoscope. Because there is a relatively fixed outer diameter available for the insertion tube, the space taken up by the transducer in an ultrasound scope (for instance) will leave less space for something else (like the working channel). Please read carefully the specifications on each bronchoscope when considering a purchase as each scope may not have the same options available.

Ease of Use

With the development of endoscopic specialization and the requirement of the operators to participate in more complex procedures, it is not unusual to spend long periods of time performing procedures. Concerns regarding operator fatigue have led to improvements in scope design. Some of these include improved maneuverability with a "rotary" function that turns the entire control body with the turn of a dial and allows it to be locked in place. In addition, some models have increased the angulation of the bending section for easier access into difficult airways.

Improved Patient Safety

Proper reprocessing of multiple use equipment such as bronchoscopes have never been more important, as more and more drug resistant organisms are being detected in patients today. Scope manufacturers are addressing these issues by trying to minimize the areas that have been traditionally hard to clean. Many scopes utilize single use, disposable biopsy, and suction valves and some have gone as far as producing bronchoscopes that can be steam sterilized. As an alternative to a sterilizable scope, there is also a bronchoscope that can be fitted with a sterile sheath over it to minimize the risk of cross infection from the equipment.

In addition, some scopes have an internal electronic scope identification system which allows you to track scope use to patient procedures. This could be very important should you need to track scope usage to a particular patient for either infection control purposes or other concerns related to the equipment.

Specialization

EBUS

Today's endoscopist may find it necessary to use more than one scope during a procedure as there are specialized bronchoscopes designed for specific functions. One that has gained much popularity is the endobronchial ultrasound scope (EBUS). This scope has a dedicated function to visualize structures below the surface of the airway by utilizing an ultrasound transducer which is part of the distal tip of the scope.

Some effects in the optics that were the result of placing the transducer in the distal tip of the scope have been addressed in recent design changes of some scopes to allow for a more forward view of the airways.

Peripheral Access Scopes

Another version of a specialized scope would be a narrow outer diameter scope that can be used to navigate to peripheral sections of the lungs but has a working channel still large enough to pass devices used to sample these areas. This type of scope has become popular in the pulmonologists armentarium as more peripheral lesions are detected today.

Portable Scopes

Tremendous improvements have been made to the technology behind portable scopes available today. These battery operated instruments do not require additional hardware such as a processor, light source, or monitor, have good illumination come with small built in monitors allowing multiple people to view and can even capture still images and video.

The Video Processor

The primary purpose of the video processor is to process the electrical signals that are produced by the video chip in the bronchoscope so that they can be read by the video monitor. There are other functions that the processor is responsible for which fine tune the image. Some are manual that the operator has control over, and others are done based on feedback that the processor has interpreted as needing adjustment.

Some manual adjustments are as follows:

- White balance control: This function, which should be performed prior to each procedure, adjusts the color that was created by the video chip to accommodate the color of the light source ... in other words, it teaches the processor to understand that the color white is really white.
- Image color adjustment: This allows fine tuning of the colors but should be made only after the white balance function is performed.
- Iris settings: This is a manual adjustment that is usually used in the "average" mode, but can be changed to "peak" mode to view areas that appear washed out.
- Image enhancement: This gives the operator the ability to enhance the image to meet his or her needs.
- Some automatic adjustments include:
- Auto-focus: Depending on the depth of the field, the system adjusts for the distance to the object to provide focusing without manual adjustments.

- Automatic brightness control: This automatically adjusts the light to the airway to maintain a constant level of brightness even if the distance changes from the end of the scope to the object being viewed.

Other options that an operator has control over through the video processor controls are:

- Video freeze, capture, enlargement, picture in picture, and other programming
- The ability to access scope history, the number of uses, and scope serial number
- The ability to save images to a video capture card in the event that there is not a computer or printer attached

Most video processors are compatible with scopes produced during that "generation," but are also compatible for scopes of recent generations as well (backward compatibility). This is important for facilities that are adding new scopes and processors to their inventory. Their older scopes are still able to function in the newer processor.

This can be important in a situation when multiple scopes may be needed during a single procedure, and one of the scopes is from a different generation (very common). Imagine the difficulty of having to change processors and all the cables to the monitor just to use a different scope.

This is of course a big advantage when you need to add a scope during a single procedure, but is also very useful when performing procedures in different locations as is the case nowadays as many endoscopists perform procedures in their procedure suite and depending on the acuity of the situation, also perform procedures in the operating room.

Most of these other locations have their own video towers and at times all that is needed is to bring the particular scopes to that location. This saves not only on the time to transport all that equipment, but on the wear and tear and potential damage of moving expensive equipment.

Integration of the Bronchoscope with Other Components of the System to Create the Video System

Correct integration of the flexible bronchoscope with the other components of the bronchoscopy system is critical to proper visualization of the image and cannot be taken lightly. The operators need to ensure that the system is functioning properly prior to the examination and, whether they rely on their own internal support or an outside department (such as clinical engineering), there needs to be a system in place to correct for any issues that may arise during a procedure during which one cannot afford to lose an image at a critical time. Refer to manufacturer's instruction manual for specific applications.

There are many configurations that one can use to route the image from the bronchoscope to the video monitor, but generally the information flows from the camera in the bronchoscope through the video processor to the video monitor. Peripherals such as video recorders can get their feeds either before or after the monitor. The way the image is transmitted to the video monitor depends on the outputs in the video processor, but can include a variety of sources such as composite, super video (S-video); red, green, blue (RGB), or (in some later processors) serial digital interface/digital video interface (SDI/DVI). It is critical for the operator to realize that the quality of the image on the monitor is only as good as its weakest link. In other words, you may be spending unnecessary money for a high-definition monitor if your cameras (i.e., bronchoscopes) are not of similar quality.

Proper Care of the Flexible Bronchoscope

This section is by far the most important part of this chapter. The price of the average bronchoscope today costs well over $20,000. This equipment is not only expensive to purchase, but very expensive to repair. In a busy program, the cost of repairs can exceed $100,000 per year; although many of these repairs can be prevented. One of the best ways to prevent damage is to read and follow the instruction manual for each instrument.

In order to provide a systematic approach to the care of the bronchoscope, this section is divided into three parts to distinguish between how to care for the equipment during different aspects of the bronchoscopy procedure.

Pre-procedure Care of the Bronchoscope

Items to consider before the procedure include:

1. Transportation of the instrument to the procedure area: Transport the scope from the storage area to the bronchoscopy suite in something that will protect it from damage and dust (i.e., a covered plastic bin)
2. A pre-procedure check of the systems

   a. Plumbing: Do the valves work and are channels clear?
   b. Mechanical: Does the bending section flex the proper amount and in the right direction?
   c. Electrical: Are all power systems functioning: processor, light source, and monitor?
   d. Image: Do you get a crisp image with good color?

3. Proper preparation for the operator

   a. Proper lubrication of scope: Oil-based lubricants can degrade the rubber sheath; water-based lubricants are recommended.
   b. Make sure that the cables coming from the processor to the scope are not twisted. The processor is intended to come from the left of the patient; otherwise, the cables will drape over the patient and put undue stress on the instrument.

Intra-procedure Care of the Bronchoscope

1. Proper use of:

   a. Bite blocks: Probably the single most costly "preventable" form of damage is from not using a bite block in patients who are thought to be adequately sedated.
   b. Sedation: As above.
   c. Accessories
      Scope manufacturers have placed much more effort in development of their own accessories than in the past. This is much more important now with the specialization of scopes and may help in protecting these valuable instruments from damage as they may prove to be more compatible.

      i. When placing accessories through the working channel, make sure that they are in the closed or "sheathed" position until they are visualized at the distal end.
      ii. If at any time visualization of the accessory is lost, immediately close or resheath the accessory and retract it into the working channel to prevent damage to the patient and/or the bronchoscope.

    iii. Never force an accessory through the working channel, or perforation of it can occur.

    iv. When retracting an accessory from the bronchoscope, always close or resheath the accessory.

    v. If the accessory device becomes stuck in the working channel, slowly remove the bronchoscope from the patient and then attempt to remove the device, keeping the angulation in the straight position.

2. Having an extra set of eyes

As the operator has his or her eyes focused on the video monitor, it is easy to lose track of how the bronchoscope is being held or manipulated. The assistant needs to be cognizant of this and point out if the scope is being bent too acutely and suggest a correction.

Post-procedure Care of the Bronchoscope

1. Initial cleaning at bedside:

    a. Wipe down insertion tube with wet gauze

    b. Flush water through scope with only the very tip submerged

    c. Suction air through for at least 10 seconds

2. Transport to cleaning area in a leakproof container that is supported on the bottom (i.e., transport tray).

3. Leak testing

    a. Apply leak test before submersing fully in water to prevent fluid invasion

    b. Flex control lever for several seconds while under water to detect minute leaks

    c. Observe for sufficient period of time

4. Proper disinfection, drying, and storage: Follow manufacturer's recommendations for scope reprocessing.

Damage to the Bronchoscope

Occasionally, or sometimes not occasionally, damage will occur to the bronchoscope. The person responsible for overseeing the service should determine the cause of the damage. It's important to distinguish between damage considered preventable in the hands of a careful operator versus damage that happens irrespective of the care that the operator takes in handling the equipment.

Preventable damage to the bronchoscope occurs when operators of the equipment or their assistants perform maneuvers that are not recommended with either the bronchoscope or its accessories. Simply stated, if one follows the manufacturer's recommendations, essentially most of this damage would not happen. Examples of this type of damage include:

- Inadequate sedation to patient resulting in bites on the instrument.
- The improper use of accessories damaging the working channel. When using devices like biopsy forceps, brushes, or needles, care should be taken to ensure that the sampling devices are not open during passage through the working channel of the instrument.

This is by far the most common reason for damage to the channel of the scope and is completely preventable.
- Improper transportation of the instrument leading to damage.

Non-preventable damage is caused by the normal wear and tear of the instrument. Examples of this type of damage include:
- Leaks in the bending section without obvious trauma during a procedure
- The degree of angulation of the bending section is out of specifications from stretching of cables

Post-damage Considerations

When damage does occur, one needs to consider how to deal with it. There are many questions that need to be addressed before deciding what to do. Here are some items to consider:
- Type of damage (this will help indicate the cost of repair)
- Age of scope
- History of repairs
- Is the scope under warranty? (Damage is not covered if it is from a preventable incident)

After you have this information, you can better make a determination as to whether or not to repair the instrument. At some point in the life of the scope, one needs to consider whether it is financially reasonable to repair it or whether it should be retired. This may be a scope whose useful life has expired a while ago, and you were hoping to just get another six months out of it before replacing it. If the decision is to retire the scope, there may still be some value in using it as a trade-in for a replacement.

If the decision is to repair it, there are many options to consider. Some of them may be:
- Who can repair it? Manufacturer versus third party?
- What is the cost of the repair?
- What is the turnaround time for the repair? You may not be able to go without having this scope for very long.
- Are there loaner scopes available?
- What are the service warranties for the repair?

Prevention of Future Damage

The first step to take in prevention of future damage is to look historically at what types of damage have occurred in the past. Therefore, it is imperative to have a system in place that tracks the damage to the instrument with the type of procedure performed (including tracking those individuals performing the procedure). There needs to be a way to associate the scope used on a patient with the staff performing the procedure. (There are other infection control reasons to be able to track patients with the scope being used, but that does not pertain to this discussion). A simple logbook of repairs should be kept for each scope sent out for service. This will give you information so that when that scope is damaged in the future, then informed decisions can be made as to what the financial feasibility is for the repair.

When determinations have been made as to why damage has taken place, a plan should be developed to prevent future damage. This plan could be relatively simple, like protecting the scope from trauma during transportation, or could involve additional training of staff to make them aware of the idiosyncrasies of a particular accessory that tends to lead to damage.

Further Readings

Culver D, Minai O, Gordon S, Mehta A. Infection control and radiation safety in the bronchoscopy suite. In: Wang K, Mehta A, Turner J, eds. *Flexible Bronchoscopy*. 2nd ed., Vol. 3. Malden, MA: Blackwell Publishing; 2004:9–25.

Gilbert CR, Akulian JA, Feller-Kopman D, Yarmus L. Ergonomics and Bronchoscopy: a survey of the American Association of Bronchoscopy and Interventional Pulmonology. *J Bronchology Interv Pulmonol*. 2013;20(2):113–120.

Ikeda S, Yanai N, Ishikawa S. Flexible bronchofiberscope. *Keio J Med*. 1968;17:1–16.

Karl Stoz Endoscopy-America Inc. Non-Invasive Troubleshooting of Endoscopic Video Systems. Karl Storz Endoscopy-America Inc., Culver City, CA, 1999.

Kirkpatrick MB, Smith JR, Hoffman PJ. Bronchoscope damage and repair costs: results of a regional postal survey. *Respir Care*. 1992;37:1256–1259.

Lee FYW. Care and maintenance of the flexible bronchoscope. In: Feinsilver SH, Fein AM, eds. *Textbook of Bronchoscopy*. Baltimore: Williams and Wilkins; 1995:100–108.

Lunn W, Garland R, Gryniuk L, Smith L, FellerKopman D, Ernst A. Reducing maintenance and repair costs in an interventional pulmonology program. *Chest*. 2005;127:1382–1387.

Mehta AC, Curtis PS, Scalzitti ML, Meeker DP. The high price of bronchoscopy. Maintenance and repair of the flexible fiberoptic bronchoscope. *Chest*. 1990;98:448–454.

Mehta A, Prakash U, Garland R, et al. American College of Chest Physicians and American Association for Bronchology Consensus Statement. Prevention of flexible bronchoscopy-associated infection. *Chest*. 2005;128:1742–1755.

Olympus America Inc. How to Prevent Instrument Malfunctions for Gastrointestinal and Bronchial Endoscopes. Olympus America Inc., Center Valley, PA, 2004.

Olympus BF-1T180 (Evis Bronchoscopy Systems Operation Manual) Olympus America Inc., Center Valley, PA, 2007.

Olympus CV-180 (Evis Bronchoscopy Systems Operation Manual). Olympus America Inc., Center Valley, PA, 2007.

Prakash UBS. Bronchoscopy unit, expertise, equipment and personnel. In: Bollinger CT, Mathur PN, eds. *Interventional Bronchoscopy. Progress in Respiratory Research*. Vol. 30. Basel: Karger; 2000:31–43.

Rivera MP, Mehta A, Wahidi MM. Establishing the diagnosis of lung cancer. *Chest*. 2013;143(5)(suppl):e142S–e165S.

Stelck M, Kulas M, Mehta A. Maintenance of the bronchoscope and bronchoscopy equipment. In: Prakash U, ed. *Bronchoscopy*. Vol. 28. New York: Raven Press; 1994:381–391.

Starting and Managing a Bronchoscopy Unit

Rabih Bechara

Interventional Pulmonology and the practice of pulmonary endoscopy have evolved tremendously in the past decade. Thanks to new technology, the trained pulmonologist can now perform a large array of diagnostic and therapeutic interventions. Importantly, the complexity of these procedures demands training, and national standards should be met before performing them. In addition, it is clear that the success in these procedures depends only partly on the skills of the physician; the skills of the support staff and the adequacy of the facilities and related resources are also indispensable. Regulating agencies such as Departments of Public Health Services, Joint Commission, and The Health Insurance Portability and Accountability (HIPAA) have released rigorous standards affecting work and workflow in endoscopy units in general. Although pulmonologists are frequently in charge of bronchoscopy units, they are generally not prepared during a fellowship to manage these units. In fact, starting or directing a bronchoscopy unit requires substantial knowledge of the necessary staff, equipment, training, procedure, space, and applicable regulations and legislation. To help provide this knowledge, I briefly describe these requirements here and comment on their importance in ensuring the success of bronchoscopic services.

The Intake and Recovery Area

A dedicated intake and recovery area should be available where nurses can receive and prepare patients for procedures and to help them recover after procedures (Figures 7.1a,b and 7.2). Here, patients will have their medical records updated and their medications verified to be sure the procedure can be performed safely. Each patient has his or her own space in the intake and recovery area, with spacers to provide privacy. In each dedicated personal space, the patient can change into the appropriate attire for the procedure, receive an identifying wrist band, have an intravenous line established, and have a place to store personal belongings safely (for example, any loose dental appliances, jewelry, just to name a few). It is important to note that all discussions and interactions between the patient and healthcare providers in the intake/recovery areas are performed with utmost respect and privacy. Each patient space is equipped to monitor vital signs and oxygen saturation. Suction and oxygen outlets are also indispensable. Further, it should be sufficient to allow patients to be placed on the bed or stretcher appropriate for their procedure (for instance, fluoroscopy, electromagnetic navigation, brachytherapy, etc...). The intake and recovery area should have at least one negative-pressure isolation room for patients who require such management. Importantly, the patient's name, attending physician, and procedures to be performed should be clearly displayed, and the status of the patient and the procedure should be monitored at all times, either electronically or on a schedule board. The latter is performed with the utmost respect to patient's privacy regulations. Transportation to

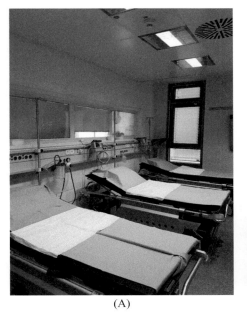
(A)

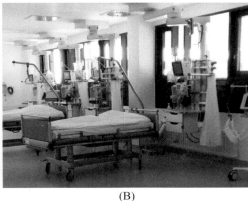
(B)

Figure 7.1 (A) An intake area in a bronchoscopy suite. **(B)** A recovery area in a bronchoscopy suite.

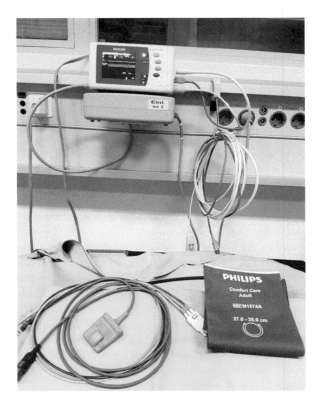

Figure 7.2 An individual patient space in an intake and recovery area showing monitors and a mobile workstation. Note that adequate dividers secure privacy.

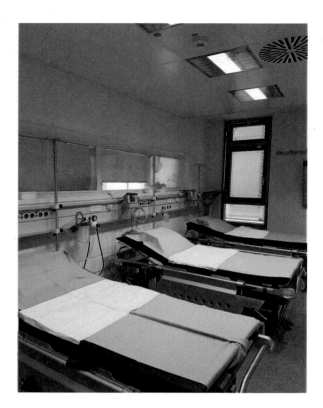

Figure 7.3 Hallways from the intake and recovery area to procedure rooms should always be kept clear.

and from the intake and recovery area, especially to the procedure suites should be direct and without interruption; hallways should be free from clutter and competing foot traffic (Figure 7.3).

The Bronchoscopy Procedure Room

Procedure rooms should be large enough to accommodate the equipment and staff needed to perform a specific procedure. As a general rule, room size ranges between 500 and 800 square feet. Note that rooms dedicated to more complex procedures may require more space than others. In all cases, there must be room for two individuals to stand at the head of the patient's bed, and the patient must be accessible from all sides at all times. Lighting must be sufficient and easily dimmed to maximize viewing quality during procedures. Because the electrical connections on bronchoscopes are on the left side, the processors and other equipment are usually positioned on the left side of the patient's bed, to allow easy access and to decrease potential clutter at the work site during procedures. It is advisable that bronchoscopes are stored in a nearby central location easily accessible (Figure 7.4). After use, they should be routed immediately to a disinfection/sterilization room, which is ideally located in the endoscopy suite for easy access. Procedure rooms should also have enough space to store the equipment needed during procedures, such as tubes, slides, special media, stents, balloons, chest tubes, etc... The locations of each item should be clearly labeled for ease of retrieval. Emergency resuscitation equipment and carts should be easily accessible, and their storage locations in the endoscopy suite should be common knowledge to all staff.

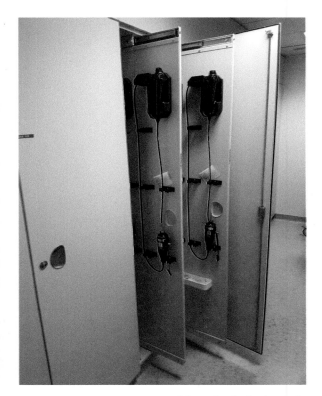

Figure 7.4 Bronchoscopes can be stored in the procedure room or in a nearby central location.

Viewing monitors are accessible to both the bronchoscopist and the assistant. If possible, monitors should be adjustable, to allow maximum flexibility in lateral direction, height, and rotation. The number of monitors per patient varies among different centers, but each room should have at least two (Figure 7.5). Rooms are also equipped with oxygen outlets, suction devices, sinks, and hand hygiene supplies. In general, procedure rooms should be ventilated with negative-pressure air exchanges, and fluoroscopy rooms (for C-arm biplanar machines) need to be able to store protective coverings for the staff (Figure 7.6).

In rooms where specimens are prepared for rapid on-site evaluation, the work area should be free of clutter and be equipped to allow specimens to be processed promptly during the procedure. The latter includes a microscope, slides, and appropriate preparation solutions. In some facilities, advanced surgical procedures are performed in bronchoscopy rooms; therefore, they need adequate overhead surgical lighting and sterile equipment (Figure 7.7). Measures to maintain the sterility of the surgical field should also be easily implemented. In such rooms, space for general anesthesia equipment must also be available. All procedure rooms should have easy access to resuscitation equipment, including airway boxes for endotracheal intubations. Cardiac defibrillators should be located in each room or in a nearby central location. In procedure rooms, access to medical records and radiographic records is crucial. Proceduralist should have capacity to display this information in monitors prior and during their procedures. The experience that a patient has from a procedure is largely dictated by external factors, rather than the endoscopic intervention. Proper sedation, a generally pleasant atmosphere, and minimized chatter and loud noises during procedures are signs of a professional endoscopy unit.

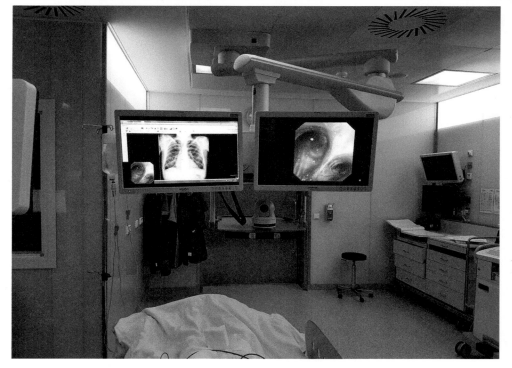

Figure 7.5 A basic bronchoscopy suite showing two endoscopy monitors.

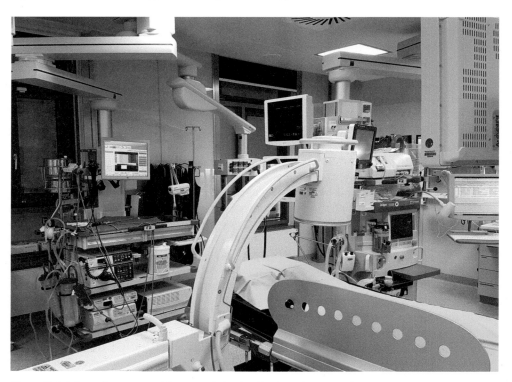

Figure 7.6 A C-arm fluoroscope with an appropriate bed in a bronchoscopy suite.

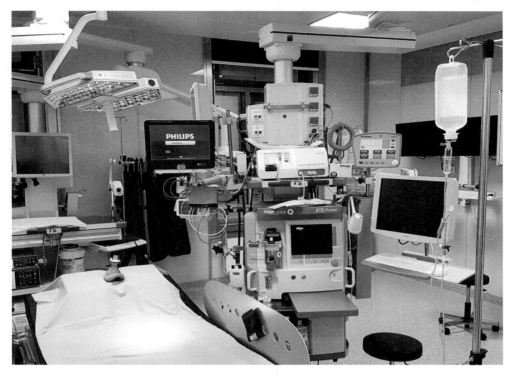

Figure 7.7 Advanced bronchoscopy room includes surgical light, adequate monitors, and anesthesia equipment.

Workstations

Proper documentation, by dictation and image, is important both for patient management and communication, and for accurate billing. Thus, endoscopy suites should have dedicated workstations separate from the procedure rooms. These stations should include computers, special forms, dictation equipment, monitors, printers, and so on, and are important for completing procedure-related paperwork. Patient-related endoscopic information should be easily available at each workstation.

Endoscopy Assistants

Endoscopy assistants have important duties before, during, and after every procedure. In fact, they are very important persons in the suite: The success of the procedures depends greatly on their training, skill, and dedication. They are responsible for preparing the room, the equipment, and patients for each procedure and for handling the specimens and used equipment after the procedure.

Bronchoscopy Equipment

Bronchoscopy requires a variety of equipment for performing specific diagnostic and therapeutic interventions. Equipment acquisition should thus be determined by the kind, extent, and complexity of the procedures to be undertaken in the unit. Diagnostic airway procedures and, occasionally, minimally invasive pleural procedures are common, and require the resources described further. Several manufacturers make several different kinds of flexible bronchoscopes. Generally, all these scopes are adequate for examining the tracheobronchial tree. They range in size from ultrathin and pediatric scopes, to those with diameters of 5.3 mm and working channels of 2.0 mm for adults, to therapeutic scopes with working channels of 3.2 mm. Other equipment include endoscopic ultrasonography (linear and radial), peripheral navigation systems, just to name a few. In some endoscopy suite Cone Beam Computerized Tomography equipment is utilized for accurate localization of targets during peripheral navigation procedures. All equipment must be stored in identified areas, and not placed in hallways. Importantly, some rooms have to be electromagnetically mapped prior to procedures. In units where gastrointestinal endoscopies are also performed, gastrointestinal endoscopes must be separated from bronchoscopes at all times, especially during processing, cleaning, and storage. In addition, labeling each scope and keeping accurate records of each are essential.

Fluoroscopy

Fluoroscopy is often useful in performing bronchoscopic procedures, including trans-bronchial biopsies, electromagnetic navigation, and a variety of routine pleural interventions. Radiation exposure from the recently introduced digital pulse fluoroscope is substantially lower than that from traditional fluoroscopes. When choosing a fluoroscopic system, remember that biplanar systems are more accurate than single-planar systems. Computed tomographic fluoroscopy is also available. In any case, all personnel in the fluoroscopy suite must wear dosimetry badges, and in many institutions, nonradiologists must pass a basic examination on fluoroscopic safety.

Therapeutic Endoscopy Equipment

Therapeutic endoscopy equipment includes, but is not limited to, cryoprobes, cryoballoons, lasers, electrocautery, argon plasma coagulation, and airway stents. This equipment should be available in suites where therapeutic techniques, such as those for managing patients with obstructed airways, with hemoptysis secondary to endobronchial lesions, and candidates for photodynamic therapy, are performed. These patients are usually high risk; therefore, staff education and preparation should be appropriate to ensure success. In addition, comprehensive support from thoracic surgery is mandatory, especially for managing complications requiring surgical interventions.

The Diagnosis and Management of Pleural Disease

In recent years, pulmonologists have become more involved in diagnosing and managing patients with pleural effusions, from both malignant and nonmalignant causes. Some minimally invasive pleural procedures and, more recently, invasive pleural procedures are being performed in bronchoscopy units. Thoracic ultrasonography has recently emerged as a standard in imaging pleural effusions because the risk of complications during thoracocentesis is greatly reduced. Fortunately, these systems are portable and can be used in other areas as well as in bronchoscopy units. Pleuroscopes are now available for performing invasive pleural interventions. These semi-rigid scopes allow visual examination and biopsy of the pleural space, and the light sources and processors are the same as those used for bronchoscopes.

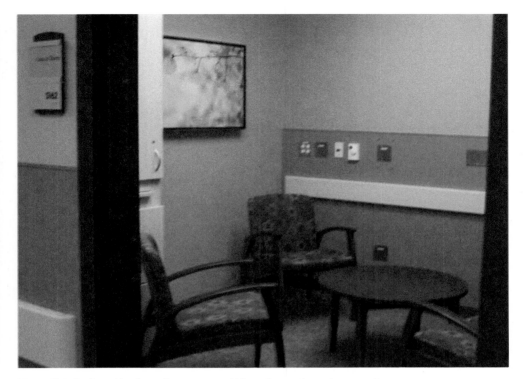

Figure 7.8 Dedicated family conference room within or close to the endoscopy suite.

Family Conference Rooms

It is a standard practice to update family members on the status of their loved ones after procedures are performed. Such discussions are not performed in public waiting areas, but in dedicated conference rooms within or close to the endoscopy suite (Figure 7.8). The latter assures confidentiality and privacy.

Summary

In summary, planning a bronchoscopy unit depends on the kinds of diagnostic and therapeutic procedures to be performed. The procedures dictate the equipment, personnel, and training necessary to perform them. Given the high risk of some patients, a comprehensive and collegial relationship with thoracic surgery is essential. The importance of staff training and preparation in the safety and success of the bronchoscopy unit cannot be overstated.

Further Readings

Bandoh S, Fujita J, Tojo Y, et al. Diagnostic accuracyand safety of flexible bronchoscopy with multiplanar reconstruction images and ultrafast Papanicolaou stain: evaluating solitary pulmonary nodules. *Chest.* 2003;124(5):1985–1992.

Beamis JF Jr. Interventional pulmonology techniques for treating malignant large airway obstruction: an update. *Curr Opin Pulmon Med.* 2005;11(4):292–295.

Bechara RI, Parks C, Ernst A. Electromagnetic navigation endoscopy. *Future Oncology*. 2011;7(1): 31–36.

Haas AR, Sterman DH, Musani AI. Malignant pleural effusions: management options with consideration of coding, billing, and a decision approach. *Chest*. 2007;132(3):1036–1041.

Herth FJ, Eberhardt R, Ernst A. The future of bronchoscopy in diagnosing, staging and treatment of lung cancer. *Respiration*. 2006;73(4):399–409.

Hohenforst-Schmidt W, Zarogoulidis P, Vogl T, Turner JF, Browning R, Linsmeier B, Huang H, Li Q, Darwiche K, Freitag L, Simoff M, Kioumis I, Zarogoulidis K, Brachmann J. Cone Beam Computertomography (CBCT) in interventional chest medicine – high feasibility for endobronchial realtime navigation. *Journal of Cancer*. 2014;5(3):231–241.

Jain P, Pleming P, Mehta A. Radiation safety for healthcare workers in the bronchoscopy suite. *Clin Chest Med*. 1999;20(1):33–38.

Jurado J, Saqi A, Maxfield R, Newmark A, Lavelle M, Bacchetta M, Gorenstein L, Dovidio F, Ginsburg ME, Sonett J, Bulman W. The efficacy of EBUS-guided transbronchial needle aspiration for molecular testing in lung adenocarcinoma. *Annals of Thoracic Surgery*. 2013;96(4):1196–1202.

Kern L, Robert J, Brutsche M. Management of parapneumonic effusion and empyema: medical thoracoscopy and surgical approach. *Respiration*. 2011;82(2):193–196.

Mathur PN, Loddenkemper R. Medical thoracoscopy. Role in pleural and lung diseases. *Clin Chest Med*. 1995;16(3):487–496.

Shulman L, Ost D. Advances in bronchoscopic diagnosis of lung cancer. *Curr Opin Pulmon Med*. 2007;13(4):271–277.

Silvestri G, Feller-Kopman D, Chen A, Wahidi M, Yasufuku K, Ernst A. Latest advances in advanced diagnostic and therapeutic pulmonary procedures. *Chest*. 2012;142(6):1636–1644.

Strack L, Brawner E, Bruns A, Devulapally K, McCullers M, Phillips G, McCallister J. Delays and efficiency in the bronchoscopy suite: perception meets reality. *Journal of Bronchology & Interventional Pulmonology*. 2010;17(3):209–217.

Chapter 8

Flexible Bronchoscopy: Indications, Contraindications, and Consent

Aaron B. Waxman

Introduction

The ability of the flexible bronchoscope to provide either diagnostic data or a therapeutic intervention is changing with technology. Improvements in digital imaging and materials along with newer interfaces utilizing global positioning technology and diagnostic imaging are enhancing the capabilities of flexible bronchoscopy. Thus the role of flexible bronchoscopy in practice is changing and will depend on the facilities available at a particular center. This review covers the broad indications and the relatively few contraindications for flexible bronchoscopy based on the current state of the art. The considerations for obtaining informed consent as it pertains to flexible bronchoscopy will also be reviewed.

Indications for Flexible Bronchoscopy

Indications for flexible bronchoscopy are often thought of in terms of diagnosis and therapy. For diagnostic bronchoscopy we can divide areas broadly into endobronchial signs and symptoms, findings from diagnostic studies such as chest radiography, and those based on specific injuries that may impact the airways. Symptoms and signs of endobronchial disease are the most common indications for flexible bronchoscopy and include chronic cough, hemoptysis, focal unexplained atelectasis with or without a fever, or a post obstructive pneumonia. In the setting of suspected complicated infection, flexible bronchoscopy combined with lavage, washings, and protected specimen brushings can be used to obtain specific cultures and cells for microbiologic analysis. Because of the directional control that flexible bronchoscopy provides cultures can be obtained from specific segments of the lung based on radiographic guidance.

Findings on exam can also be indications for flexible bronchoscopy including a localized wheeze, which could be the result of something partially blocking an airway. Patients with what sounds like refractory "asthma" or focal findings of wheezing on examination, or altered breath sounds associated with a radiographic finding may be appropriate indications (Figure 8.1). Patients who have abnormal flow volume curves may have obstructing lesions in the large airways that can easily be assessed using a flexible bronchoscope. While stridorus breath sounds may be considered a tempting indication for taking a look, any patient with stridor needs to be approached with great caution and with a well-planned approach to the difficult airway. Findings that can cause changes in examination of the chest or respiratory symptoms might include an endobronchial neoplasm, broncholithiasis, stricture or stenosis of large airways, foreign body aspiration, extrinsic compression of an airway by a parenchymal or mediastinal tumor or lymph node, a bronchopleural fistula, paradoxical vocal cord dysfunction, or the carcinoid syndrome. Very often an abnormal chest radiograph will result

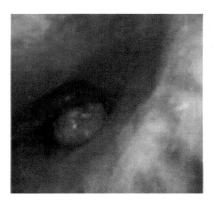

Figure 8.1 Broncholith in a patient with a persistent focal wheeze on physical examination in spite of maximal therapy for asthma.

in a referral for flexible bronchoscopy. Findings that raise concern and are indications for flexible bronchoscopy include an obvious mass lesion, or a recurring pulmonary infiltrate in the same anatomical region that may signal an obstructive lesion (Figure 8.2). Persistent atelectasis could signal a compressive lesion or endobronchial obstruction due to a tumor or foreign body. Mediastinal abnormalities such as enlarged lymph nodes that are abutting the trachea and accessible by transtracheal or transbronchial needle biopsy may be seen on chest radiograph or computed tomography of the chest. Likewise diffuse parenchymal disease such as sarcoidosis may be approached with the bronchoscope for a diagnosis (Figure 8.3). In other cases of interstitial lung disease, flexible bronchoscopic sampling may not provide enough tissue for a definitive diagnosis and thoracoscopic or open lung biopsy may still be required.

One of the most important indications for bronchoscopy is in the diagnosis of lung cancer. The bronchoscope can be used to make a tissue diagnosis via endobronchial, transbroncial, or needle biopsy; for staging of lung cancer with transtracheal lymph node biopsy; or early

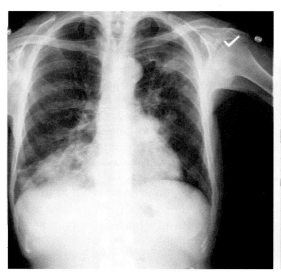
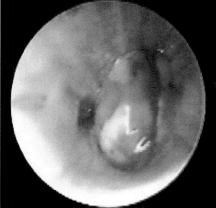

Figure 8.2 Chest radiograph from patient with recurrent pneumonia. Bronchoscopy revealed an obstructive lesion in the right lower lobe.

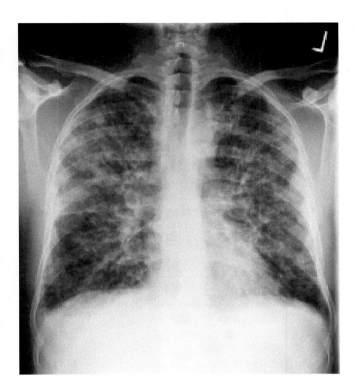

Figure 8.3 Diffuse lung disease that on transbronchial biopsy was consistent with sarcoidosis.

diagnosis in the setting of chronic cough or abnormal chest radiograph in the appropriate patient.

Patients who suffer traumatic injuries may require bronchoscopy in order to assess the extent of injury. This might include patients who have suffered extensive burn or thermal injury and are suspected of having injuries to the lower airways. Because these patients may have significant debris or tissue damage, diagnostic bronchoscopy may be combined with therapeutic bronchoscopy for purposes of rinsing out debris or necrotic tissue. Likewise patients who have suffered blunt or penetrating thoracic trauma may require bronchoscopy to assess for bronchial disruption or fracture. Finally, in the intensive care unit in patients who are intubated, bronchoscopy can be utilized for assessment of endotracheal tube position.

Therapeutic bronchoscopy covers a number of areas. One of the more important and often difficult indications for flexible bronchoscopy is in the removal of a foreign body. In general, foreign body removal is best done with a rigid bronchoscope under general anesthesia. Flexible bronchoscopy can be used as an initial screening procedure for suspected cases of aspiration. Patients with known or suspected foreign bodies should undergo rigid bronchoscopy. If the evidence for aspiration is equivocal, patients should undergo diagnostic flexible bronchoscopy. If a foreign body is found, a rigid bronchoscopy can follow. In certain cases, a foreign body extraction can be done using a flexible bronchoscope, but this is often a rare case.

When a patient presents with lung abscess flexible bronchoscopy can be performed to rule out endobronchial obstruction as a result of foreign body or a mass lesion. In certain cases the bronchoscope can be used for drainage of the abscess cavity. Other indications may include tracheal stenosis requiring dilation and possible stenting, or refractory atelectasis that may benefit from a balloon dilatation.

Occasionally, flexible bronchoscopy will be indicated for respiratory toilette. As a general rule, postural drainage, cough, and suction of secretions are sufficient. If for some reason these cannot be done, then bronchoscopy can be done for respiratory toilette. Prospective studies have shown that good intensive respiratory toilette can accomplish good results in the control of atelectasis. However, there are many clinical circumstances when respiratory toilette cannot ideally be accomplished. These include immobilized patients, patients with spine or spinal cord injury, patients with thoracic trauma such as flail chest or postoperative patients where pain is a significant issue, or patients supported with an aortic balloon pump. Some bronchoscopists advocate treating left lower lobe atelectasis with the flexible bronchoscope and lavage. In general blind passage of a mini BAL catheter or blind suctioning in the intubated patient with in line catheters are hard to direct to specific regions such as the left lower lobe. In cases where it is important to verify where a sample is obtained, flexible bronchoscopy provides obvious benefit.

Flexible bronchoscopy may serve as a prelude to other procedures or interventions. In patients with pneumonia or diffuse lung disease, bronchoscopy can be done to obtain respiratory secretions for establishing the diagnosis of an infection. The choice of brushing, protected brush specimen, or broncho-alveolar lavage is dependent on the clinical situation and can be done following airway inspection.

If you experience difficulty in performing an intubation, or anticipate a difficult intubation a flexible bronchoscope can be used. The endotracheal tube is placed over the flexible bronchoscope and once the bronchoscope is advanced through the vocal cords and is in a good position, the endotracheal tube is passed over the bronchoscope and, under direct vision, can be introduced into the trachea and it's position verified.

There are a number of conditions in which flexible bronchoscopy may not be helpful. This is dependent on the state of available technology and the experience of the bronchoscopist. An important example is the peripheral solitary pulmonary nodule beyond the reach of the bronchoscope (Figure 8.4). Further, there is no role for bronchoscopy in the setting of an isolated pleural effusion, or a chronic cough in a patient who is younger than 55, with a clear chest radiograph, and no smoking history or risk factors for lung cancer. Acute stridor in children is a medical emergency and an absolute contraindication for bronchoscopy. In cases of uncomplicated pneumonia, either community acquired or hospital acquired pneumonia, bronchoscopy often adds little information and has no impact on medical decision-making. Lastly, in cases of massive hemoptysis, the flexible bronchoscope is often too small and ineffective in clearing blood fast enough to prevent occlusion of the airway or to find and treat a source of bleeding. Rigid bronchoscopy is the preferred approach to massive hemoptysis.

Contraindications to Flexible Bronchoscopy

To date there have not been any trials to assess those factors that may increase the risk for patients undergoing flexible bronchoscopy. The decision to perform flexible bronchoscopy, like any procedure, must be made after weighing the potential benefits of the procedure against the potential risk to the patient. In general most contraindications to flexible bronchoscopy are relative rather than absolute and are based on common sense. There should be available to the bronchoscopist adequate facilities and personnel to care for emergencies

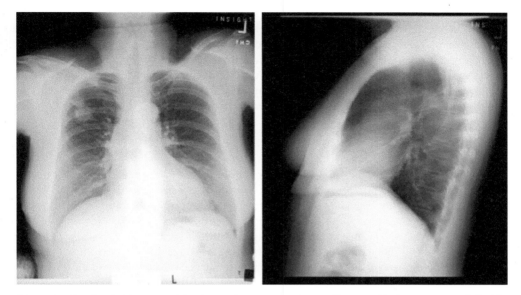

Figure 8.4 Peripheral right upper lobe lesion that may not be readily accessible by conventional flexible bronchoscopy.

that could occur during the procedure including cardiopulmonary arrest, pneumothorax, or bleeding. An inability to adequately oxygenate the patient during the procedure based on their clinical presentation is a clear contraindication to performing bronchoscopy, particularly in a non-intubated patient. When assessing a patient before the procedure, special attention must be paid to the patient's respiratory status and the patient's potential for clinical decline as a result of the procedure. This might include patients with severe obstructive airways disease, patients with severe refractory hypoxemia, or patients with an unstable hemodynamic status. Like wise, assessment of a patient's bleeding status is critical, especially when biopsies are being considered. The procedure may need to be postponed in a patient whose coagulopathy or bleeding diathesis cannot be corrected.

Relative contraindications to this, or any procedure, might include lack of patient cooperation, a recent myocardial infarction or unstable angina, a partial tracheal obstruction, moderate-to-severe hypoxemia, or hypercarbia. Depending on available facilities and comorbidities additional relative contraindications might include morbid obesity or severe sleep apnea. It is preferable that patients do not undergo elective conscious sedation until 8-hours after a solid meal or 2–4 hours after clear liquids or medications given orally.

Hazards and Complications of Flexible Bronchoscopy

Even though flexible bronchoscopy is a relatively safe and well tolerated procedure, there are still a number of potential complications. Complications can include airway problems including those that result from irritation including laryngospasm, increased airway resistance and exacerbation of obstructive airways disease, and physical obstruction. There can be mechanical problems including epistaxis, hemoptysis, or pneumothorax. Complications can be directly hemodynamically important such as cardiac arrhythmias including brady-cardia, or other vagally mediated phenomena, tachyarrhythmias, or cardiac arrest. The bronchoscopes themselves can pose a hazard to both the bronchoscopist and the patient through exposure to infection. Cross-contamination of specimens or bronchoscopes has also occurred. In general flexible bronchoscopy is usually an extraordinarily safe procedure with major complications such as, bleeding, respiratory depression, and pneumothorax occurring in less than 1 percent of cases. Mortality is rare, with a reported death rate of 0 to 0.04 percent in a large number of procedures.

Consent and Pre-screening

When obtaining consent start out with a clear explanation of the procedure. Make an example of the size of the bronchoscope with a finger, or show the patient the actual bronchoscope, to allay their anxieties. Everyone fears suffocation and gagging so it is important to assure the patient that there is sufficient room for air to go through the throat while the scope is in their airway. Explain how the gag reflex and gagging are alleviated, in most cases, with topical lidocaine. This will also help to decrease coughing. Make it clear to the patient that the scope is going to pass through their vocal cords and that they should try not to talk during the procedure as it can cause damage to the vocal cords. Recall that there is no pain sensation within the lung; only the pleura are innervated with pain fibers, so the patient should not feel any pain during a flexible bronchoscopy. The response to irritation in the lung is to cough and we suppress the cough with topical anesthetics. Work out hand signals so that the patient can let you know how they are doing or can answer any questions without talking.

Prior to the procedure we do a pre-procedure screen that includes obtaining a history of allergic reactions to local anesthetic. If clinically indicated we will check BUN (>30mg/dL) and creatinine (>3.0 mg/dL), platelet count (<50K), PT and PTT, especially if biopsies are being considered. If indicated, a complete blood count should also be checked. In appropriate circumstances we will evaluate for evidence of a recent MI or active cardiac issues. There should be an evaluation of American Society of Anesthesiologists (ASA) class and a proper airway assessment such as the Mallampatti grade or equivalent. In many centers patients graded as an ASA III or higher are required to have an electrocardiogram within the last six months or if there are risk factors for myocardial disease. Everyone is encouraged to review their center specific protocols before administering conscious sedation.

Informed Consent

Informed consent is obtained for all therapeutic and diagnostic procedures. In all cases the patient, or a patient's surrogate, should give consent voluntarily. Regardless of who is giving consent, the patient or their proxy, you should be certain they are competent to provide con-sent. It is a good practice that the information about the procedure is provided by a person who is participating in the procedure. Consent should be worded in plain English (or with the assistance of an appropriate interpreter) at no more than an eighth grade reading and com-prehension level. In every case you should clearly explain the rationale, the inherent risks, the potential benefits for the procedure, and any alternatives to the procedure (Box 1). Con-sent should be obtained prior to any sedation being given to the patient. Once the patient is under sedation they may misinterpret or forget what you say. When discussing the procedure with the patient, make it clear to them that they should not expect results right away. Micro-biologic results can take days to weeks before results are available. Cytology and pathology

Box 1 Suggested Wording of Potential Complications While Explaining the Risks of Flexible Bronchoscopy to a Patient

- Low blood oxygen
- Difficulty breathing that might require oxygen, assisted breathing, or admission to the intensive care unit
- Adverse drug reaction
- Abnormal heart rhythm
- Fever
- Infection
- Sore throat
- Air leak around the lung with lung collapse
- Death

evaluation can take several days for tissue processing and evaluation before results can be available.

Further Readings

Borchers SD. Beamis JF. Jr. Flexible bronchoscopy. *Chest Surgery Clinics of North America.* 6(2):169–92, 1996 May.

de Blic J. Marchac V. Scheinmann P. Complications of flexible bronchoscopy in children: prospective study of 1,328 procedures. *European Respiratory Journal.* 20(5):1271–6, 2002 Nov.

Herth FJ. Eberhardt R. Ernst A. The future of bronchoscopy in diagnosing, staging and treatment of lung cancer. *Respiration.* 73(4):399–409, 2006, April.

Kreider ME. Lipson DA. Bronchoscopy for atelectasis in the ICU: a case report and review of the literature. *Chest.* 124(1):344–50, 2003 Jul.

Mazzone P. Jain P. Arroliga AC. Matthay RA. Bronchoscopy and needle biopsy techniques for diagnosis and staging of lung cancer. *Clinics in Chest Medicine.* 23(1):137–58, 2002 Mar.

Pryor JA. Physiotherapy for airway clearance in adults. *European Respiratory Journal.* 14(6):1418–24, 1999 Dec.

Chapter 9

Bronchial Washing, Bronchoalveolar Lavage, Bronchial Brush, and Endobronchial Biopsy

Melissa Tukey and Carla Lamb

Introduction

Bronchial washings (BWs), bronchoalveolar lavage (BAL), bronchial brushings, and endobronchial biopsies (EBBX) are common bronchoscopic sampling techniques used by clinicians for the evaluation and management of infectious and non-infectious pulmonary pathology. Often there is a complementary role between these sampling modalities, which can also be combined with transbronchial needle aspiration (TBNA) and transbronchial lung biopsy (TBBX) in the appropriate clinical context. This review provides the bronchoscopist with a practical guide to procedural decision making including specimen collection, diagnostic approach, and individual procedural risks. The indications and contraindications for flexible bronchoscopy in general are discussed in another chapter.

When approaching the patient with an abnormal chest radiograph or computed tomography (CT) scan, it is important to plan a strategy of questions to be answered and specimens collected well before the bronchoscopic procedure even begins. It is worthwhile to create a broad differential diagnosis based on the patient's history specifically in terms of immunocompetence, medication and environmental exposures, infectious contacts, and travel. Risk factors for malignancy should also be assessed. Chest imaging will identify the extent and location of disease. These variables will be used to determine the bronchoscopic tests to be ordered and the location of the samples to be obtained as well as the quantity of specimen required. Communication with the bronchoscopy team is essential to ensure the preparation of the proper tools for specimen retrieval and collection as well as appropriate respiratory isolation of the patient and staff in specific clinical settings. Communication with the microbiology and the cytology departments is also important. Listing a patient's specific differential diagnosis when completing the cytology lab request forms will improve the cytopathologic review by alerting the pathologist to your clinical concerns.

Bronchial Washings

Collection of BWs most often occurs in conjunction with other sampling modalities such as bronchial brushings and EBBX for the diagnosis of primary or metastatic pulmonary malignancy. BWs must be distinguished from the more standardized BAL. In comparison to BAL, BWs do not require wedging of the bronchoscope into a subsegmental position and the volume of saline flushed into the desired bronchial site is far less, ranging from 5 to 50 mL. Generally 5–15 mL of fluid will be required for basic microbiologic evaluation and 10 mL for cytology. Although BWs can be used for diagnosis of infection, true bacterial quantification for diagnosing pneumonia is limited because of both specimen size and the high potential for large airway respiratory flora contamination. For these reasons BAL is considered superior to BW for the diagnosis of pulmonary infection.

The literature is conflicting as to whether the addition of BWs to bronchial brushings and EBBX increases the overall diagnostic yield in patients with endoscopically visible tumors. While some recommend that BWs should be performed prior to bronchial brushings or biopsies to avoid contamination of the specimen with red blood cells obscuring cytologic interpretation, recent literature suggests similar diagnostic yield of BWs performed before and after biopsies and brushings. It should be noted that acute infection may create atypical squamous metaplasia that can be nearly impossible to differentiate from malignancy and thus cytology performed on BWs should be interpreted with caution and in the appropriate clinical context.

Bronchoalveolar Lavage

BAL allows for the sampling of cellular and non-cellular alveolar contents and is considered a standard diagnostic tool in the setting of both infectious and non-infectious pulmonary disease of unknown cause. BAL is typically performed during flexible bronchoscopy under local anesthesia and moderate sedation or through an endotracheal tube in ventilated patients. In general there are no absolute contraindications to BAL other than those otherwise associated with flexible bronchoscopy. BAL is generally well tolerated even in critically ill patients. The most frequent complication is fever, which is typically self-limited. BAL may be associated with transient worsening hypoxemia which is particularly relevant in critically ill patients with tenuous oxygen saturations who may require increased ventilatory support post-procedure. In comparison to other bronchoscopic sampling modalities, particularly transbronchial lung biopsy, the risk of clinically significant bleeding associated with BAL is minimal.

Despite the widespread use of BAL there is no consensus regarding the optimal technique to be used. In patients with diffuse disease, the right middle lobe or lingua are preferred as the percentage of instilled fluid that is recovered is higher than when the lower lobes are selected. Alternatively, in patients with localized abnormalities or marked radiographic heterogeneity it is recommended that BAL be performed in the area of greatest abnormality. During standard flexible bronchoscopy, BAL is performed after inspection of the airways but before other sampling techniques to decrease the risk of contamination of the sample. The tip of the bronchoscope is advanced into the selected bronchopulmonary subsegment until a "wedge" position is obtained. The wedge position should be at the level of the third or fourth order bronchi (Figure 9.1). The wedge position is confirmed by noting slight collapse of the distal airway with application of gentle suction, while avoiding "over-wedging" which can cause trauma to the airway mucosa, reduce recovery volume, and alter the fluid profile by adding blood. Once the wedge position is obtained, isotonic sterile saline is instilled through the working channel of the bronchoscope in 20- to 60-mL aliquots. Although not standardized, the total volume instilled is generally between 100 and 300 mL divided into three to five aliquots. After instillation of each aliquot the fluid is recovered either by manually aspirating through the working channel of the bronchoscope using an attached 20 mL syringe or by applying gentle wall suction into a sterile collection trap. A recovery of 40–70 percent of the instilled volume is considered normal. Ideally suction should be minimized while passing through the nasopharynx and central airways prior to BAL and the amount of lidocaine flushed through

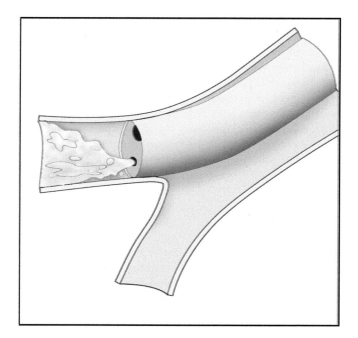

Figure 9.1 Wedge position of the bronchoscope for BAL in the third- to fourth-order subsegmental bronchi. (Illustration by Carla Lamb and Vinald Francis.)

the working channel prior to specimen collection limited as both can alter the cellular yield of the specimen. Some bronchoscopists advocate discarding the first "bronchial" aliquot to avoid contamination of the following "alveolar" aliquots. The BAL fluid should be collected in silicone or plastic containers that do not promote adhesion of cellular material to the container surface.

Specimen handling and processing from the bronchoscopy suite to the microbiology and cytology labs are as important as the methods of collection during the procedure. Ideally specimens should be processed within 1–4 hours of collection or refrigerated if a delay is anticipated. BAL fluid should be transferred on ice or at room temperature if it can be processed within an hour of collection. The exact volume of fluid required for specific tests can be variable but generally 40–60 mL return fluid is adequate to run most desired tests. For a more detailed review of specimen processing technique, see suggested readings.

Knowledge of the range of cellular findings in normal individuals is necessary to assess the adequacy of sampling as well as to define pathologic findings. Cellular contents in BAL of normal controls consist of approximately 90 percent macrophages, 5 percent lymphocytes, and 0–5 percent neutrophils, eosinophils or basophils. Paucity of epithelial cells and erythrocytes is desired. An unsatisfactory sample may be defined as the lack of alveolar macrophages, excessive airway epithelial cells (>5 percent), or an abundance of purulent material from the central airways.

The role of BAL in the evaluation of pulmonary disease is best described in terms of specific disease entities. Some general indications for BAL include diffuse alveolar or interstitial lung disease, unresolving pneumonia, alveolar hemorrhage, abnormal imaging in the immunocompromised host, diagnosis of ventilator associated pneumonia and other infections, and malignancy. The bronchoscopist should be aware of the studies that can be sent on a BAL sample (Table 9.1). BAL may be used as a stand-alone test for diagnosis of a number

Table 9.1 Studies for BW, BAL, Bronchial Brush, and EBBX

BW/BAL	Brush	EBBX
AFB/modified AFB (Kinyoun)	AFB	AFB
Fungal stains/culture	Fungal	Fungal
Bacterial (quantitative)	Bacterial Clt (Quant)	Bacterial Clt
Viral	Viral	Viral
Legionella (DFA/Clt)		
Silver stain for *Pneumocystis*		
PCR for tuberculosis		
DFA for *Pneumocystis*		
Galactomannan for *Aspergillus*		
Cell count and differential		
CD4-to-CD8 ratio		
Cytology	Cytology	Cytopathology
Flow cytometry (cell markers)		Flow cytometry (for lymphoma)

Note: AFB, acid-fast bacilli; Clt, culture; DFA, direct fluorescence antibody; PCR, polymerase chain reaction.

of infectious and non-infectious lung diseases. Although the presence of certain findings is definitive in some disease entities, other findings may not correlate directly with actual disease and their presence must be interpreted in the clinical context of the patient (Tables 9.2–9.4). The key is to approach the patient with a strategy of the type of analysis to be performed, decide if BAL alone will answer the diagnostic question, review chest images to determine site of collection, adhere to a standardized technique, and confirm wedge position through the procedure.

Table 9.2 Role of BAL in Infectious Disease States

If Identified in BAL	
Pathogenic	**Use Clinical Context May Not Be Pathogenic**
• Bacteria predominant 10,000 cfu/mL	• *Aspergillus*
• *Histoplasma capsulatum*, Blastomyces, Coccidioidomycosis	• Atypical *Mycobacterium*
• Influenza	• *Candida*
• *Legionella*	• *Cryptococcus*
	• Cytomegalovirus
	• Herpes simplex
• *Mycobacterium* tuberculosis	
• *Mycoplasma*	
• *Pneumocystis jiroveci*	
• Respiratory syncytial virus	
• *Strongyloides* (other parasitic organisms)	
• *Toxoplasma gondii*	

Adapted from: *Am J Respir Crit Care Med.* 1990;142:481–486.

Table 9.3 Role of BAL in Noninfectious Diseases

Diagnostic	Suggestive, No Definitive
Pulmonary alveolar proteinosis	Alveolar hemorrhage
Langerhans cell histiocytosis	Asbestosis
Lipoid pneumonia/Fat embolism	Berylliosis
Malignancy	Drug-induced disease (amiodarone)
	Eosinophilic pneumonias
	Hypersensitivity pneumonitis
	Sarcoidosis
	Silicosis

Adapted from: *Am J Respir Crit Care Med*. 1990;142:481–486.

Role of Bronchoalveolar Lavage in Disease-Specific Entities

Ventilator-Associated Pneumonia

Ventilator-associated pneumonia (VAP) is a disease process in which BAL may have a specific role not only to assist with identification of a pathogen but also to rule out other non-infectious causes of airspace disease in the critically ill patient with respiratory failure. Lower respiratory tract sampling is appropriate in any critically ill patient with an abnormal CXR who is suspected of having VAP. Lower respiratory tract samples may be obtained either by non-bronchoscopic or bronchoscopic techniques. Non-bronchoscopic lower airway tract sampling techniques include blind tracheobronchial aspiration and "mini-BAL" during which a catheter is inserted through the endotracheal tube until resistance is met and subsequently sterile saline is instilled through the catheter and aspirated. Bronchoscopic

Table 9.4 Disease Associations with BAL Studies/Findings

Microbiologic	Cytologic
KOH: fungal	Sulfur granules: actinomyces
India ink: *Cryptococcus*	Hemosiderin-laden macrophages (alveolar hemorrhage) >20% red blood cells
Modified acid fast: *Nocardia*	Foamy macrophages: amiodarone, alveolar proteinosis, *Pneumocystis*
Ziehl-Neelsen, Auramine O: *Mycobacteria*	Malignancies
Silver methenamine: *Pneumocystis*/fungal	Oil Red O stain: fat embolism
Gram stain: predominant bacterial	Sudan stain: lipoid pneumonia >20% eosinophils: acute or chronic eosinophilic pneumonia, allergic bronchopulmonary aspergillosis, Churg–Strauss toxic inhalation, drug reaction
	Increased CD4-to-CD8 ratio: sarcoidosis, berylliosis, asbestosis, connective tissue disease
	Decreased CD4-to-CD8 ratio: hypersensitivity pneumonitis, silicosis, drug-induced disease, rheumatoid disease
	Periodic acid–Schiff: alveolar proteinosis
	Flow cytometry: lymphoma

lower airway tract sampling can be performed by BAL or protected specimen brush (PSB), which will be discussed later in this chapter. In general non-bronchoscopic lower airway tract sampling has been found to be as successful as the more invasive bronchoscopic methods. Bronchoscopy is performed at a greater expense, requires trained personnel, and has not been shown to have an impact on mortality or hospital length of stay, however, may allow for de-escalation of broad-spectrum antibiotics. The decision to perform bronchoscopic or non-bronchoscopic sampling therefore should be made in a case by case basis.

If BAL is to be performed as part of the evaluation of VAP, collection of specimens prior to initiation of antibiotics or within 48 hours of antibiotics is recommended. Avoiding inadvertent contact of the bronchoscope tip to the external environment of the patient is also important to avoid contamination of the instrument. VAP is defined with quantitative BAL cultures of 10,000 colony-forming units (cfu) per milliliter of a predominant pathogen (or if there is strong clinical suspicion 1,000–10,000 cfu/mL). Semiquantitative cultures, which are typically reported as light, moderate, or heavy growth, can also be performed on BAL specimens. While quantitative and semi-quantitative BAL cultures have been shown to have a similar impact on clinical outcomes there is a greater risk of false-positive results with semi-quantitative culture techniques.

Fungal Pneumonias

The presence of *Histoplasma capsulatum*, *Blastomyces dermatitidis*, or *Coccidioides immitis* signifies pathogenesis when present in BAL fluid. Although often considered a pathogen, *Cryptococcus neoformans* can colonize the airway in some instances and must be interpreted in the context of the individual patient. Fungal organisms can be detected on gram stain and silver stain along with fungal cultures.

Although the presence of *Aspergillus* in BAL fluid may not represent pathogenicity in all cases, in the appropriate clinical context of an immunocompromised host in the critical care setting it should strongly be considered. Assessing for invasive aspergillus is necessary. The sensitivity of BAL culture and microscopy for the diagnosis of invasive pulmonary aspergillosis has been estimated to be approximately 50 percent. An additional study sometimes used to identify invasive fungal disease is BAL galactomannan. Galactomannan is a polysaccharide present in the cell wall of most *Aspergillus* species that is released during invasion into the patient's tissues. Galactomannan can be detected in body fluids including BAL using a sandwich-type ELISA. Of note, exposure to beta-lactam antibiotics can cause a false positive result. The clinical usefulness of BAL galatcomannan remains unclear. While the diagnostic accuracy of BAL galactomannan is considered superior to serum galactomannan, the overall performance of BAL galactomannan described in the literature has been highly variable with reported sensitivities and specificities ranging from 50–100 percent and 73–95 percent respectively.

Mycobacterium Tuberculosis

In patients who are unable to expectorate a sputum sample or in whom sputum induction with hypertonic saline is non-diagnostic, bronchoscopy with BAL is recommended. Bronchoscopy should always be performed using appropriate respiratory protective equipment in an environment with negative pressure relative to adjacent areas. In patients who are able to undergo successful sputum induction, the addition of BAL has not been shown to increase diagnostic yield. While the yield of BAL AFB-smear in patients with smear-negative induced

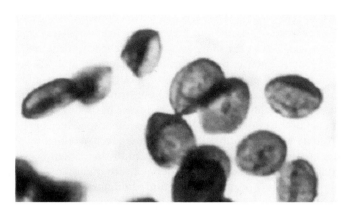

Figure 9.2 *Pneumocystis jiroveci* as seen in BAL specimen with silver stain.

sputum samples is low, cultures may be positive in over 70 percent of cases. The addition of BAL fluid nucleic acid amplification testing (NAAT) may also improve diagnostic yield in smear-negative patients and help to distinguish non-tuberculous mycobacterial disease from tuberculous disease when the AFB smear is positive. In patients suspected of having military tuberculosis, sputum AFB smears are typically negative and if bronchoscopy is performed the addition of transbronchial lung biopsies should be considered.

Tropical Pneumonias

There is a wide range of pathogens and diseases that make up the tropical infectious pneumonias. Bronchoscopy with BAL may be helpful in a number of these, which include *Burkholderia pseudomallei* (melioidosis, nocardiosis, *Cryptococcus neoformans*, tuberculosis, coccidioidomycosis, paracoccidioidomycosis, *Syngamus laryngeus* (syngamosis), hookworm, paragonimiasis, amebiasis, *Echinococcus*, filariasis, *Strongyloides*, ascariasis, and toxoplasmosis.)

Immunocompromised Host

BAL is a useful tool for the evaluation of pulmonary infiltrates in the immunocompromised host including patients with HIV and both hematopoietic and solid-organ transplant recipients. Given the broad range of both infectious and non-infectious disease processes that can affect the immunocompromised patient, in general, an aggressive approach to the evaluation of pulmonary infiltrates is recommended. One exception may be the neutropenic patient with acute respiratory failure in the intensive care unit in which the routine use of diagnostic BAL infrequently leads to a change in treatment compared to non-invasive testing. In the immunocompromised patient, BAL is often complementary to bronchial brushings and transbronchial lung biopsies.

An organism that deserves special mention in the immunocompromised population is *Pneumocystis jiroveci* (Figure 9.2). BAL sensitivity exceeds 90 percent and it is always a pathogen when it is found in bronchoalveolar fluid. It may be more difficult to identify this organism beyond 10–15 days into a treatment course and in patients receiving prophylactic therapy with aerosolized pentamidine. Since pneumocystis cannot be cultured, diagnosis relies on visualization of the organism in respiratory specimens. While pneumocystis organisms can be identified by general stains such as Diff-Quik (Baxter Diagnostics, Inc, McGaw

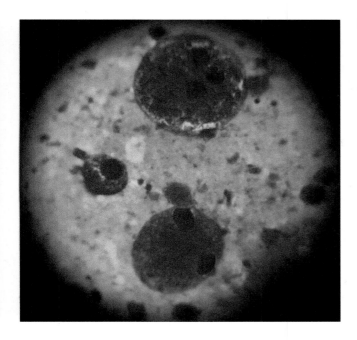

Figure 9.3 Alveolar macrophages filled engorged with PAS-positive material in PAP.

Park, IL) or methenamine silver, direct fluorescent antibody (DFA) staining is the most sensitive and is considered the gold standard.

Pulmonary Alveolar Proteinosis

BAL plays a significant role in the diagnosis of pulmonary alveolar proteinosis (PAP). The hallmark of PAP is the deposition of periodic acid–Schiff (PAS) positive proteinaceous material within the alveolar spaces and in and around alveolar macrophages (Figure 9.3). The diagnosis is suggested by the appearance of milky material with sediment on BAL, and is confirmed with a positive PAS stain from either BAL or transbronchial lung biopsy. When performing bronchoscopy with BAL in adults with suspected PAP it is important to look for possible secondary causes of PAP including hematologic malignancy, *Nocardia*, *Pneumocystis*, and viral infections. In patients with moderate to severe symptoms, the treatment of choice is whole lung lavage. In contrast to BAL, whole lung lavage is performed under general anesthesia using a double lumen endotracheal tube and lavage volumes of 1 to 1.5 liters of warm saline are instilled until lavage effluent clears (typically a total of 10 to 15 lavages are required).

Interstitial Lung Disease

BAL may be helpful in the evaluation of patients with suspected interstitial lung disease based on chest imaging, however, it is generally not diagnostic as a stand-alone test. If the decision is made to perform BAL in a patient with suspected interstitial lung disease, a differential cell count should be performed in addition to standard microbiologic and cytologic testing. The predominance or absence of certain inflammatory cells in the BAL cell count can help narrow the differential diagnosis in the evaluation of diffuse interstitial disease when high resolution CT scan features are non-diagnostic. For example the predominance of eosinophils supports the diagnosis of eosinophilic pneumonia or drug reactions, while BAL lymphocytosis is commonly seen in hypersensitivity pneumonitis, sarcoidosis, pneumotoxic drug reactions, and cellular NSIP. In contrast, the absence of prominent BAL lymphocytosis or eosinophilia supports the diagnosis of idiopathic pulmonary fibrosis. BAL cellular analysis has not consistently been correlated with prognosis in interstitial lung disease and is not clearly predictive of response to therapy.

Eosinophilic Lung Disease

The cell count and differential obtained from BAL maybe helpful in limiting the differential diagnosis in patients with diffuse lung disease. While mild to moderate BAL eosinophilia (i.e., <25 percent) can be seen in a number of diseases including interstitial pulmonary fibrosis, fungal pneumonias, drug induced lung disease, and sarcoidosis, very high BAL eosinophil counts (i.e., ≥25 percent) suggest a diagnosis of acute eosinophilic pneumonia, chronic eosinophilic pneumonia, eosinophilic granulomatosis, and polyangiitis (i.e., Churg–Strauss syndrome) or tropical pulmonary eosinophilia.

Diffuse Alveolar Hemorrhage

Bronchoscopy with BAL plays an important role in the evaluation of patients with diffuse alveolar hemorrhage. To diagnose alveolar hemorrhage, the bronchoscope is wedged in the desired subsegment and sequential aliquots of approximately 50 mL sterile saline are instilled and retrieved without breaking wedge position. The diagnosis of alveolar hemorrhage is confirmed by the retrieval of macroscopically bloody BAL fluid that becomes increasingly hemorrhagic from fraction to fraction. On BAL microscopy, the presence of hemosiderin-laden macrophages also indicates alveolar hemorrhage. While BAL can confirm the diagnosis of alveolar hemorrhage, it has limited utility in differentiating between the many potential etiologies.

Langerhans Cell Histiocytosis

Pulmonary Langerhans Cell Histiocytosis is a rare interstitial lung disease that typically presents in young adults and is highly associated with smoking. On CT scan both cysts and nodules with a mid to upper lobe predominance are seen. The pathologic cell type is the Langerhans cell which can be identified in BAL fluid by its pale cytoplasm, large nucleus and nucleoli, and positive staining for CD1a and S-100. The Langerhans cell is also characterized by the presence of Birbeck granules on electron microscopy, however, this is often not performed due to cost. The presence of > 5 percent Langerhans cells on BAL differential cell count is strongly suggestive of the disease. It is important to note, however, that lower proportions of Langerhans cells can be seen in patients with other types of interstitial lung disease and in healthy smokers.

Sarcoidosis

BAL alone is not sufficient as a sole diagnostic procedure for sarcoidosis as the presence of non-caseating granulomas is necessary for diagnosis. Nevertheless, as an adjunct to endobronchial and transbronchial lung biopsies, certain BAL findings may enhance the diagnostic sensitivity of bronchoscopy. In sarcoidosis, the BAL cell count typically demonstrates a lymphocytic predominance. If sarcoidosis is suspected based on clinical and radiographic findings, a lymphocyte subset analysis, which evaluates the ratio of activated T-helper cells (CD4$^+$ cells) to T-suppressor cells (CD8$^+$), can be performed to aid in the diagnosis. While the CD4/CD8 ratio is highly variable in sarcoidosis and its use for diagnostic purposes is controversial, the combination of BAL lymphocytosis in addition to a CD4/CD8 ratio $\geq$4:1 demonstrates a positive predictive value of 94 percent for sarcoidosis. Conversely if the CD4/CD8 ratio is <1:1, the negative predictive value has been reported to be 100 percent.

Berylliosis

As in sarcoidosis, a BAL lymphocytosis and increased CD4/CD8 ratio may be seen in chronic beryllium disease. BAL cells may be used in beryllium lymphocyte transformation testing to assist in this diagnosis.

Asbestosis

The finding of asbestos bodies in BAL indicates exposure but does not directly correlate with the presence of disease. Their presence, however, may be helpful in identifying occupational exposure and those who may be at increased risk for asbestosis.

Hypersensitivity Pneumonitis

BAL may support the diagnosis of hypersensitivity pneumonitis by demonstrating often marked BAL lymphocytosis as well as a decreased CD4-to-CD8 ratio of <1:1.

Drug-Induced Lung Diseases

Many drugs have been associated with pulmonary toxicity. Generally, this group of diseases demonstrates mixed cellularity on BAL differential. Amiodarone toxicity may demonstrate "foamy macrophages" in BAL fluid because of phospholipid accumulation. The presence of foamy macrophages in the patient on amiodarone serves as a marker for exposure, but the findings need to be correlated with radiographic and physiologic changes to define true amiodarone-related lung disease.

Malignancy

The diagnostic yield of BAL for malignancy can be 69 percent or greater in the presence of visible endobronchial disease. BAL is also considered a highly effective method to obtain cytologic proof of lymphangitic carcinomatosis. BAL is often recommended to be performed prior to biopsies to reduce the obscuration of diagnostic cytologic cells by erythrocytes. Atypical cells can be seen in the setting of acute inflammation and should be interpreted with caution and in the clinical context of the patient.

Bronchial Brushing

Bronchial brushings can be obtained for microbiologic analysis or to assist in the diagnosis of malignancy. There is a selection of brushes (3-mm and 7-mm bristles) that can be used for specimen collection (Figure 9.4). The brush should be kept within its protective sheath while it is passed through the working channel of the bronchoscope channel, and then directed to the target site as an assistant advances the brush out approximately 3 cm or so from the

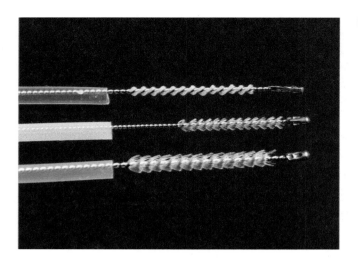

Figure 9.4 Bronchial brushes of varying sizes for microbiologic and cytologic evaluation.

tip of the bronchoscope. Vigorous brush strokes are then applied to the lesion. Communication to the assistant to bring the brush into its sheath when specimens have been retrieved should occur before the sheath and brush are pulled back through the working channel. Distal bronchial brushings or transbronchial brushings are usually performed with fluoroscopic guidance so as to avoid breaching the pleura and potentially causing a pneumothorax. In the setting of lung cancer with visible endobronchial disease, the yield of bronchial brushing has been reported to be between 50 percent and 90 percent. Studies have also indicated that performing bronchial brushings along with BWs and EBBX in the setting of visible endobronchial disease is cost effective. The primary complication of endobronchial brushing is bleeding, and it is best avoided in the irreversibly coagulopathic patient.

Protected Specimen Brush for VAP

The protected specimen brush (PSB) is a brush contained within a protective sheath designed to maintain sterility and avoid contamination of the brush while traversing the proximal tracheobronchial tree. Not only is this brush safely encased in its protective sheath, there is a biodegradable plug at the distal end that is ejected when the brush is advanced in the desired location within the airway. The technique employed is similar to standard bronchial brushing. The entire PSB device is advanced 3 cm or so beyond the distal tip of the bronchoscope into the desired airway and subsequently the brush is pushed out into the secretions. After specimens are collected by brushing the airway wall the brush is retracted into the inner sheath which in turn is retracted into the outer sheath and then removed from the bronchoscope. Once the PSB is removed from the bronchoscope the distal part of the catheter is wiped with 70 percent alcohol then the brush component is advanced and cut with sterile scissors into at least 1 mL of nonbacteriostatic saline. Quantitative cultures should be requested. The diagnosis of VAP in using quantitative cultures from PSB is defined as 1000 cfu/mL or 100–1000 cfu/mL in the presence of a strong clinical suspicion. Interestingly, studies comparing PSB with bronchoscopic BAL and non-bronchoscopic lower respiratory tract sampling have not consistently demonstrated a significant advantage in diagnostic yield between any of these techniques. All are considered reliable alternatives.

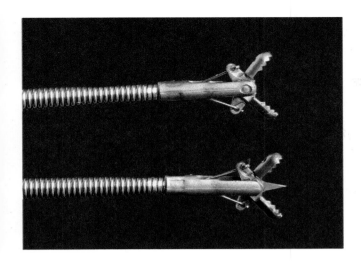

Figure 9.5 Bronchial biopsy alligator forceps without (*top*) and with (*bottom*) needle.

Endobronchial Biopsy

The technique for EBBX depends on the location of the lesion relative to the airway wall and to airway bifurcations. A "straight-on" approach is used with the biopsy forceps (either cup or alligator biopsy forceps with or without a needle) when there is a lesion that is at an airway bifurcation (Figures 9.5 and 9.6). Maintaining the bronchoscope close to the actual distal biopsy forceps and using them as one unit can provide the added leverage needed to push into the lesion to obtain a deeper core sample. If the lesion is parallel to the airway wall, then a more angular approach (preferably with the forceps with a needle) may allow for a

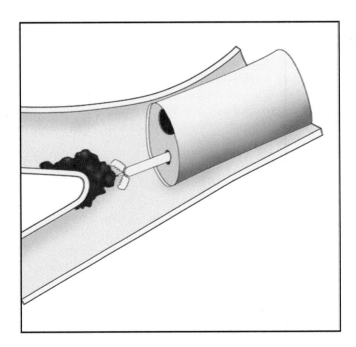

Figure 9.6 "Straight-on" approach at bronchial bifurcation with biopsy forceps with needle. (Illustration by Carla Lamb and Vinald Francis.)

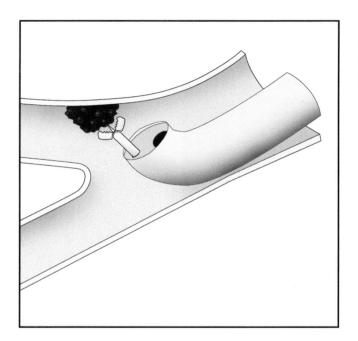

Figure 9.7 Angular side wall approach for endobronchial biopsy using needle to anchor the biopsy forceps to the tumor. (Illustration by Carla Lamb and Vinald Francis.)

more anchored position (Figure 9.7). It is advisable to take three to six biopsies in the same location to obtain material from the more central aspect of the lesion as the surface cells may represent cellular edema and necrosis and not be diagnostic. To further gain access to central diagnostic cellular material, a 19- or 21-gauge needle can be directed into the core of an endobronchial lesion.

The utility of EBBX to obtain diagnostic material is best demonstrated in malignancy and sarcoidosis. The diagnostic yield of EBBX for endoscopically visible malignant lesions has been reported to be >80 percent. In sarcoidosis, the addition of endobronchial biopsies to transbronchial biopsies has been shown to increase the yield of bronchoscopy by 20 percent. The primary complication of endobronchial biopsy is bleeding which is typically mild but can be life threatening. In general, endobronchial biopsy is not recommended in patients with uncorrectable coagulopathy, significant thrombocytopenia (platelet count <50,000), or in patients receiving clopidogrel.

Conclusions

Although some of the procedures discussed here can be diagnostic individually for a variety of diseases, they are often used collectively to improve overall yield. As part of good preprocedural planning, the clinician should keep in mind the following:

- Carefully screen patients prior to the procedure for safety and ability to tolerate the anticipated diagnostic studies. Correct coagulopathies when brushes or biopsies are planned.
- Create a differential diagnosis to anticipate the volume of specimen required for desired testing.
- Be knowledgeable of the particular tests required.

- Have a strategy of collection anatomically based on chest imaging.
- Communicate to the bronchoscopy team the anticipated studies to ensure that proper specimen media are readily available.
- Communicate to microbiology and cytopathology the history and differential diagnosis to increase the level of awareness of specific disease entities.
- Recognize the diagnostic strengths and limits of each of these diagnostic procedures.

Further Readings

Affolter K, Tamm M, Jahn K, et al. Galactomannan in bronchoalveolar lavage for diagnosing invasive fungal disease. *Am J Respir Crit Care Med*. 2014;190:309–317.

American Thoracic Society. Infectious Diseases Society of America: guidelines for the management of adults with hospital-acquired, ventilator-associated, and healthcare-associated pneumonia. *Am J Respir Crit Care Med*. 2005;171:388–416.

Anderson C, Inhaber N, Menzies D. Comparison of sputum induction with fiber-optic bronchoscopy in the diagnosis of tuberculosis. *Am J Respir Crit Care Med*. 1995;152:1570–1574.

Azoulay E, Mokart D, Lambert J, et al. Diagnostic strategy for hematology and oncology patients with acute respiratory failure: randomized controlled trial. *Am J Respir Crit Care Med*. 2010;182:1038–1046.

Azoulay E, Mokart D, Rabbat A, et al. Diagnostic bronchoscopy in hematology and oncology patients with acute respiratory failure: prospective multicenter data. *Crit Care Med*. 2008;36:100–107.

Baughman RP, Dohn MN, Loudon RG, et al. Bronchoscopy with bronchoalveolar lavage in tuberculosis and fungal infections. *Chest*. 1991;99:92–97.

Boersma WG, Erjavec Z, van der Werf TS, et al. Bronchoscopic diagnosis of pulmonary infiltrates in granulocytopenic patients with hematologic malignancies: BAL versus PSB and PBAL. *Respir Med*. 2007;101:317–325.

Bronchoalveolar lavage constituents in healthy individuals, idiopathic pulmonary fibrosis, and selected comparison groups. The BAL Cooperative Group Steering Committee. *Am Rev Respir Dis*. 1990;141:S169–202.

Brown M, Varia H, Bassett P, et al. Prospective study of sputum induction, gastric washing, and bronchoalveolar lavage for the diagnosis of pulmonary tuberculosis in patients who are unable to expectorate. *Clin Infect Dis*. 2007;44:1415–1420.

Canadian Critical Care Trials Group. A randomized trial of diagnostic techniques for ventilator-associated pneumonia. *N Engl J Med*. 2006;355:2619–2630.

Centers for Disease Control and Prevention (CDC). Updated guidelines for the use of nucleic acid amplification tests in the diagnosis of tuberculosis. *MMWR Morb Mortal Wkly Rep*. 2009;58:7–10.

Chastre J, Combes A, Luyt CE. The invasive (quantitative) diagnosis of ventilator-associated pneumonia. *Respir Care*. 2005;50:797–807.

Cole P, Turton C, Lanyon H, et al. Bronchoalveolar lavage for the preparation of free lung cells: technique and complications. *Br J Dis Chest*. 1980;74:273–278.

Costabel U, Hunninghake GW. ATS/ERS/WASOG statement on sarcoidosis. Sarcoidosis Statement Committee. American Thoracic Society. European Respiratory Society. World Association for Sarcoidosis and Other Granulomatous Disorders. *Eur Respir J*. 1999;14:735–737.

Du Rand IA, Blaikley J, Booton R, et al. British Thoracic Society guideline for diagnostic flexible bronchoscopy in adults: accredited by NICE. *Thorax*. 2013;68 Suppl 1:i1–i44.

Fujitani S, Yu VL. Diagnosis of ventilator-associated pneumonia: focus on nonbronchoscopic techniques (nonbronchoscopic bronchoalveolar lavage, including mini-BAL, blinded protected specimen brush, and blinded bronchial sampling) and endotracheal aspirates. *J Intensive Care Med*. 2006;21:17–21.

Goldstein RA, Rohatgi PK, Bergofsky EH, et al. Clinical role of bronchoalveolar lavage in adults with pulmonary disease. *Am Rev Respir Dis*. 1990;142:481–486.

Grossman RF, Fein A. Evidence-based assessment of diagnostic tests for ventilator-associated pneumonia. Executive summary. *Chest*. 2000;117:177S–181S.

Gruson D, Hilbert G, Valentino R, et al. Utility of fiberoptic bronchoscopy in neutropenic patients admitted to the intensive care unit with pulmonary infiltrates. *Crit Care Med*. 2000;28: 2224–2230.

Harris B, Lowy FD, Stover DE, et al. Diagnostic bronchoscopy in solid-organ and hematopoietic stem cell transplantation. *Ann Am Thorac Soc*. 2013;10:39–49.

Hope WW, Walsh TJ, Denning DW. Laboratory diagnosis of invasive aspergillosis. *Lancet Infect Dis*. 2005;5:609–622.

Horvath JA, Dummer S. The use of respiratory-tract cultures in the diagnosis of invasive pulmonary aspergillosis. *Am J Med*. 1996;100:171–178.

Jain P, Sandur S, Meli Y, et al. Role of flexible bronchoscopy in immunocompromised patients with lung infiltrates. *Chest*. 2004;125:712–722.

Karahalli E, Yilmaz A, Turker H, et al. Usefulness of various diagnostic techniques during fiberoptic bronchoscopy for endoscopically visible lung cancer: should cytologic examinations be performed routinely? *Respiration*. 2001;68:611–614.

Lam B, Wong MP, Ooi C, et al. Diagnostic yield of bronchoscopic sampling methods in bronchial carcinoma. *Respirology*. 2000;5:265–270.

Lamb CR, Lederman ER, Crum NF. Bronchoscopy: diagnostic and interventional approach in tropical pulmonary diseases. In: Sharma O, ed. *Tropical Lung Disease*, 2nd ed. New York: Taylor & Francis; 2006:95–115.

Lee HS, Kwon SY, Kim DK, et al. Bronchial washing yield before and after forceps biopsy in patients with endoscopically visible lung cancers. *Respirology*. 2007;12:277–282.

Levine SJ, Kennedy D, Shelhamer JH, et al. Diagnosis of Pneumocystis carinii pneumonia by multiple lobe, site-directed bronchoalveolar lavage with immunofluorescent monoclonal antibody staining in human immunodeficiency virus-infected patients receiving aerosolized pentamidine chemoprophylaxis. *Am Rev Respir Dis*. 1992;146:838–843.

Maartens G, Willcox PA, Benatar SR. Miliary tuberculosis: rapid diagnosis, hematologic abnormalities, and outcome in 109 treated adults. *Am J Med*. 1990;89:291–296.

Meersseman W, Lagrou K, Maertens J, et al. Galactomannan in bronchoalveolar lavage fluid: a tool for diagnosing aspergillosis in intensive care unit patients. *Am J Respir Crit Care Med*. 2008;177:27–34.

Meyer KC, Raghu G, Baughman RP, et al. An official American Thoracic Society clinical practice guideline: the clinical utility of bronchoalveolar lavage cellular analysis in interstitial lung disease. *Am J Respir Crit Care Med*. 2012;185:1004–1014.

Miller RF, Huang L, Walzer PD. Pneumocystis pneumonia associated with human immunodeficiency virus. *Clin Chest Med*. 2013;34:229–241.

Pingleton SK, Harrison GF, Stechschulte DJ, et al. Effect of location, pH, and temperature of instillate in bronchoalveolar lavage in normal volunteers. *Am Rev Respir Dis*. 1983;128:1035–1037.

Rennard SI, Aalbers R, Bleecker E, et al. Bronchoalveolar lavage: performance, sampling procedure, processing and assessment. *Eur Respir J Suppl*. 1998;26:13S–15S.

Ryu YJ, Chung MP, Han J, et al. Bronchoalveolar lavage in fibrotic idiopathic interstitial pneumonias. *Respir Med*. 2007;101:655–660.

Shah PL, Hansell D, Lawson PR, et al. Pulmonary alveolar proteinosis: clinical aspects and current concepts on pathogenesis. *Thorax*. 2000;55:67–77.

Shorr AF, Torrington KG, Hnatiuk OW. Endobronchial biopsy for sarcoidosis: a prospective study. *Chest*. 2001;120:109–114.

Steinberg KP, Mitchell DR, Maunder RJ, et al. Safety of bronchoalveolar lavage in patients with adult respiratory distress syndrome. *Am Rev Respir Dis*. 1993;148:556–561.

Technical recommendations and guidelines for bronchoalveolar lavage (BAL). Report of the European Society of Pneumology Task Group. *Eur Respir J*. 1989;2:561–585.

van der Drift MA, van der Wilt GJ, Thunnissen FB, et al. A prospective study of the timing and cost-effectiveness of bronchial washing during bronchoscopy for pulmonary malignant tumors. *Chest*. 2005;128:394–400.

Veeraraghavan S, Latsi PI, Wells AU, et al. BAL findings in idiopathic nonspecific interstitial pneumonia and usual interstitial pneumonia. *Eur Respir J*. 2003;22:239–244.

Wang BM, Stern EJ, Schmidt RA, et al. Diagnosing pulmonary alveolar proteinosis. A review and an update. *Chest*. 1997;111:460–466.

Willcox PA, Potgieter PD, Bateman ED, et al. Rapid diagnosis of sputum negative miliary tuberculosis using the flexible fibreoptic bronchoscope. *Thorax*. 1986;41:681–684.

Winterbauer RH, Lammert J, Selland M, et al. Bronchoalveolar lavage cell populations in the diagnosis of sarcoidosis. *Chest*. 1993;104:352–361.

Chapter 10

Transbronchial Lung Biopsy

Scott Shofer and Momen M. Wahidi

Introduction

Transbronchial lung biopsy (TBB) is a safe and effective tool useful for the diagnosis of a wide variety of diffuse and focal pulmonary diseases. TBB is regularly performed by 69 percent of practicing physicians documented in a survey of 1800 North American pulmonary and critical care physicians. This chapter describes the primary indications and contraindications to performing TBB during bronchoscopy, our approach to TBB, and methods to manage complications that may arise during or after the procedure.

Indications

Biopsy forceps commonly used for TBB via the flexible bronchoscope are generally on the order of 3 mm or smaller in any given dimension. Because of this restriction in size, tissue samples obtained via the transbronchial approach are generally 2–3 mm in any dimension. Despite the small size, TBB provides information regarding pathology that is located beyond the cartilaginous airways that may include elements of the small airways of the distal bronchial tree, the alveolar space, the vasculature, and lymphatic structures immediately surrounding the alveoli. Pulmonary diseases that require examination of larger pieces of lung tissue to assess heterogeneity or homogeneity of different regions of the involved lung (such as many of the idiopathic interstitial lung diseases) are generally not amenable to diagnosis by TBB, so consideration of video-assisted thoracoscopic lung biopsy should be pursued for patients in whom these diseases are a strong consideration. With these limitations in mind, TBB is useful for the diagnosis of a variety of interstitial, infectious, and malignant pulmonary diseases (Box 10.1).

Interstitial Diseases

TBB has a high sensitivity for the diagnosis of sarcoidosis involving the lung. Even with Stage I disease, TBB may be positive in up to 50–85 percent of patients undergoing this procedure, although yields are greater with increasing radiographic abnormality of the lung parenchyma. To optimize sampling of tissue for sarcoidosis, a minimum of four biopsies has been suggested to be collected before termination of the procedure. TBB has a high yield in other interstitial lung diseases such as Langerhans cell histiocytosis, pulmonary alveolar proteinosis, lipoid pneumonia, eosinophilic pneumonia, and drug-induced pneumonitis.

Box 10.1 Indications for TBB

- Sarcoidosis
- Langerhans cell histiocytosis
- Pulmonary alveolar proteinosis
- Lipoid pneumonia
- Eosinophilic pneumonia
- Drug-induced pneumonitis
- Pulmonary infiltrates in the immunocompromised host
- Pulmonary nodule or mass
- Lymphangitic malignancy

Infectious Diseases

Diagnosis of infectious pulmonary disease in the immunocompromised host is a common indication for TBB. Sensitivity for infectious organisms ranges from 81 to 90 percent. Bronchoalveolar lavage (BAL) is often as efficacious as TBB in detecting infectious organisms in immunocompromised patients and use of TBB has been discouraged in the most recent BTS statement on bronchoscopy except when there is substantial suspicion for tuberculosis where it is still considered to be useful for diagnosis. Nevertheless, in most series there is a small number of patients in whom the diagnosis is made by TBB but missed with BAL. In addition, compared with BAL, TBB enhances diagnostic yield for noninfectious lung disease in immunocompromised patients (an increase in yield from 31 to 40.4 percent, respectively).

Infections with *Pneumocystis jiroveci* deserve special comment. BAL generally has excellent sensitivity for *Pneumocystis* infection in the patient with advanced HIV/AIDS, particularly when combined with immunofluorescent monoclonal antibody staining. However, the sensitivity of BAL in immunocompromised hosts without HIV/AIDS may be lower. Addition of TBB to the diagnosis of *Pneumocystis* pneumonia in patients with cancer, bone marrow transplantation, or pharmacologic immunosuppression increases the diagnostic sensitivity from 82 to 92 percent.

Neoplastic Diseases

TBB is commonly used for the diagnosis of suspicious pulmonary nodules and masses. Overall, the yield of TBB for peripheral lesions is 57 percent although the yield from a specific nodule is related to size, location, and number of pieces of tissue collected. Sensitivity increases with the size of the nodule in question, with a diagnosis obtained 34 percent of the time in nodules <2 cm and 63 percent in nodules >2 cm. The presence of an airway leading to the nodule on thoracic computed tomography scan (positive bronchus sign) increases yield from 25 to 63 percent. Diagnostic yield from pulmonary nodules increases with number of pieces of tissue collected. Popovich and colleagues examined the effect of repeated sampling of peripheral pulmonary nodules by TBB. The initial biopsy had a sensitivity of 45 percent, which increased to 70 percent by the sixth sample. In malignancies with a diffuse distribution (such as lymphangitic tumor), sensitivity of TBB is generally good.

Lung Transplant Surveillance

TBB is the primary diagnostic procedure in evaluating the presence of allograft rejection in patients after lung transplantation. Although surveillance strategies differ among various institutions, most institutions perform some form of TBB-based surveillance as well as diagnostic biopsies during periods of declining lung function in transplant recipients. Sensitivity of TBB for allograft rejection has been reported to be as high as 94 percent when ten or more pieces of tissue are collected, although most institutions do not regularly collect this many samples during surveillance bronchoscopies.

Contraindications

Contraindications for TBB are similar to those for bronchoscopy in general. Absolute contraindications are few and include inability to provide informed consent, status asthmaticus, severe hypoxemia, and unstable cardiovascular conditions. Pulmonologists' perceptions of relative contraindications to TBB were examined during a survey of 158 North American respiratory physicians. Physicians' opinions were obtained regarding the safety of TBB in the presence of thrombocytopenia, pulmonary hypertension, uremia, hypoxemia, and management of anticoagulant and antiplatelet medications.

Thrombocytopenia

Approximately 70 percent of the surveyed physicians felt that a platelet count of 50,000 was adequate to perform TBB safely. Few data are available regarding bleeding complications from TBB in the thrombocytopenic patient. One series examined 24 patients with platelet count <60,000 and an average count of 30,000. Twenty of the 24 patients received prophylactic platelet transfusion prior to TBB with an incidence of significant bleeding in four patients, one of whom expired and theremaining were self-limited. Our practice has been to use a minimum platelet value of 50,000 when TBB is planned during the bronchoscopy. We have not experienced any life-threatening bleeding events related to thrombocytopenia in our practice using this criterion.

Pulmonary Hypertension

A single prospective study is available regarding TBB and pulmonary hypertension. This study examined 37 heart transplant recipients who had measurements of pulmonary pressures obtained within 72 hours of bronchoscopy. Moderate bleeding (defined as 25–100 mL of blood) was encountered in 15 percent of the 20 patients with MPAP >16 mm Hg, whereas no significant bleeding occurred in the remaining patients. No incidence of major hemorrhage occurred in any. Current recommendations from the British Thoracic Society (BTS) suggest that caution should be observed in performance of TBB in patients with elevated pulmonary arterial pressures. We have not established a pulmonary pressure at which TBB is contraindicated within our practice, and we assess each patient individually regarding the overall clinical scenario before we commit to performing TBB.

Uremia

The presence of uremia adversely affects platelet function, resulting in abnormal platelet aggregation and prolonged bleeding times and potentially increasing the risk of significant hemorrhage in patients undergoing TBB. No studies that have rigorously examined the effect of uremia on bleeding complications in TBB currently exist. Some authors have suggested that the use of recombinant arginine vasopressin may decrease the extent of bleeding in uremic patients, although examination of the surgical literature has shown mixed results. The current practice at our institution is to give recombinant arginine vasopressin at a dose of 0.3 µg/kg intravenously to all lung transplant recipients with creatinine >2.5 mg/dL 30 minutes prior to bronchoscopy. Non-lung transplant patients generally do not receive arginine vasopressin, and we have not encountered noticeably increased rates of bleeding in these patients.

Hypoxemia

No level of oxygen supplementation is currently recognized to be an absolute contraindication to TBB, although 37 percent of surveyed pulmonologists indicated that an inspired oxygen requirement of >60 percent fraction of inspired oxygen (FiO_2) was a contraindication to TBB, whereas 36 percent of the respondents found no specific O_2 requirement a contraindication. The BTS recommends supplying supplemental O_2 to keep blood oxygen saturations >90 percent to minimize the risk of cardiac arrhythmias during and following bronchoscopy. Generally, we consider electively intubating patients for bronchoscopy when oxygen supplementation is >5 L/min via nasal cannula prior to performing TBB.

Anticoagulant and Antiplatelet Agents

Use of anticoagulants and antiplatelet agents is common among patients referred for bronchoscopy. No randomized trials exist regarding the use of warfarin in the setting of TBB. The BTS recommended holding warfarin for three days prior to bronchoscopy, or providing supplemental vitamin K prior to the procedure. Current recommendations suggest that an international normalized ratio of 1.5 is a safe level for most surgical procedures. Patients anticoagulated with heparin should have this medication held for 6 hours prior to bronchoscopy and may be restarted 12 hours following the procedure. O'Donnell and colleagues addressed the use of enoxaparin as a bridge for warfarin in patients scheduled for elective surgery. Ninety-four patients received a final dose of twice-daily enoxaparin at least 12 hours prior to surgery and were found to have persistently elevated anti-Xa levels at the time of surgery. Based on these findings, it is our policy to stop therapeutically dosed enoxaparin for 24 hours prior to performing TBB, whereas enoxaparin dosed for deep vein thrombosis prophylaxis is not administered on the morning of the procedure.

Aspirin use was previously considered to be a contraindication to TBB; however, a large multicenter study has shown no difference in bleeding following TBB in 285 patients taking aspirin at the time of bronchoscopy compared with 932 patients not on aspirin. Consequently, we do not have patients hold aspirin prior to TBB.

In a follow-up study examining the effect of the antiplatelet medication clopidogrel on incidence of bleeding during TBB, significant bleeding was increased to 89 percent compared with 3.4 percent in the control group. In a small number of patients taking both aspirin and clopidogrel, the incidence of significant bleeding was 100 percent following TBB. Given the relatively long half-life of clopidogrel, our current practice is to have patients discontinue clopidogrel a minimum of 5 days prior to undergoing bronchoscopy with TBB.

Several direct oral anticoagulants (DOACs) have been approved for use in patients with atrial fibrillation and deep vein thrombosis. These agents have bleeding risk profiles similar to warfarin and other conventional anticoagulants, however, laboratory monitoring of the effects of DOACs can be difficult since many of the necessary assays are not universally available. No specific data exist regarding use of these medications in the setting of TBB, although most expert organizations agree the drugs should not be taken 24 to 48 hours prior to invasive procedures. Drug metabolism may be altered by renal and hepatic dysfunction and so the agents should be avoided for up to 5 days in patients with impaired metabolism of DOACs, or in patients with increased risk of bleeding during TBB.

Procedural Considerations

TBB

TBB is most commonly performed via flexible bronchoscopy using conscious sedation. Careful study of a prebronchoscopy CT scan is useful in determining the best pulmonary segment to access for biopsy. In diffuse pulmonary disease, use of fluoroscopy is not necessary, although the risk of significant pneumothorax may be reduced. In focal disease that is visible on chest X-ray, use of fluoroscopy during the procedure may significantly increase the diagnostic yield of the study.

After a careful airway examination is performed, the pulmonary segment of interest is intubated with the tip of the bronchoscope, and the pulmonary forceps are passed through the working channel of the bronchoscope. As the forceps are visualized entering the pulmonary subsegment, the fluoroscopy unit may be activated to visualize the forceps as they enter the distal segments of the lung (Figure 10.1). To biopsy the lung periphery, the forceps should be gently advanced in the closed position until resistance is encountered (Figure 10.2). Next, the forceps are withdrawn approximately 1 cm, and the command is given to open the forceps jaws. The forceps are then advanced halfway to the area where resistance was encountered, and the forceps jaws are closed. With the fluoroscopy unit still activated, the forceps are retracted with firm, continuous pressure to allow the biopsy specimen to be removed from the surrounding lung parenchyma. The lung parenchyma should be watched on the fluoroscopy monitor for retraction during the collection of the biopsy sample (Figure 10.1). If there is excessive resistance, or extensive retraction of the lung parenchyma during sampling, the forceps should be opened to release the lung tissue, and the biopsy procedure should be restarted. After a sample is obtained, the forceps are removed from the working channel of the bronchoscope, and the biopsy is placed in formalin.

Two schools of thought exist as to how best to manage the airway after a biopsy sample is collected. The wedge technique may be employed, where the tip of the bronchoscope is lodged firmly (wedge position) in the airway subsegment that was sampled to monitor for bleeding. It is thought that leaving the bronchoscope wedged permits control of potential bleeding by continuous suctioning to remove extravasated blood, thereby preventing soiling of the remainder of the lung. Continuous suctioning also allows the operator to assess the quantity of bleeding present, and collapsing the distal airways produces a tamponade effect. When bleeding has slowed, the tip of the bronchoscope may be withdrawn from the wedge position to allow observation of the bleeding segment and, if necessary, to facilitate repeating the wedge maneuver if the bleeding continues to be significant. The disadvantage of the wedge maneuver is that the bronchoscopist is not able to either visualize the airways due to blood obscuring the optics of the bronchoscope or assess the effectiveness of the wedge in isolating the bleeding subsegment. In the alternative strategy, the tip of the bronchoscope is withdrawn from the subsegment of interest so that the bronchoscopist can watch for welling up of blood

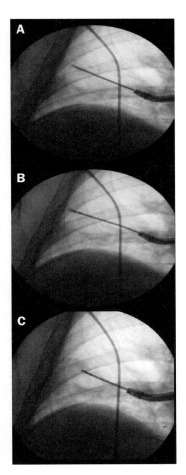

Figure 10.1 Sequence of fluoroscopic images showing TBB from the right lung. Extension of the closed biopsy forceps to the periphery of the lung **(A)**. Forceps opened and advanced to collect tissue **(B)**. Forceps closed and partially withdrawn to collect the tissue sample **(C)**. Note the subtle retraction of the underlying lung parenchyma by the forceps as the tissue sample is collected.

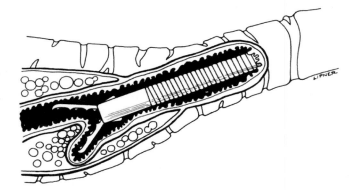

Figure 10.2 Artists representation of forceps in the distal bronchus. The jaws of the forceps produces and invagination of the bronchial wall resulting in sampling of both bronchial mucosa and alveolar tissue. (From Zavala DC. Transbronchial biopsy in diffuse lung disease. *Chest.* 1978;73:727–733, with permission.)

from the distal lung. Blood is suctioned with a back-and-forth motion to clear the airway and maintain vision. This suctioning permits a more global assessment of the extent of bleeding and potential seepage of blood into the other portions of the lung. There are currently no data to support the superiority of either approach. Our practice is to have novice bronchoscopists maintain the bronchoscope in the wedge position after each biopsy and use the observational technique after they have acquired more experience with the bronchoscope. Additional discussion of the management of bleeding complications will be presented later.

Optimizing Biopsy Yield

Forceps Biopsy

Several studies have examined how best to enhance biopsy yield in terms of number of samples to be collected and characteristics of the collected specimens. As described earlier, the number of tissue pieces needed to optimize sensitivity is dependent on the underlying disease. Most studies report a range of 4–10 pieces of tissue to optimize sampling sensitivity and the BTS guidelines on flexible bronchoscopy recommend five to six samples in patients with diffuse lung disease and seven to eight samples in patients with focal lung disease. Our practice is to obtain a minimum of six tissue pieces of a minimum size of 1–2 mm in the long axis for patients with either focal or diffuse lung disease.

Several studies have examined the optimal size of biopsy forceps for performing TBB and no clear difference has been established regarding size of tissue samples or diagnostic sensitivity between large and small forceps. Our practice is to use medium sized alligator style forceps (Figure 10.3) for all of our TBBs because they do not entirely occlude the working channel of the bronchoscope while the forceps are extended, thereby permitting continued use of the working channel for suctioning. Larger forceps show no clear advantage in biopsy quality, but do preclude effective suctioning while they are deployed.

Adjunctive Techniques for TBB

Two recent technologic advances have shown the ability to improve diagnostic yield for transbronchial lung biopsy in peripheral lesions. The first, radial probe endobronchial ultrasound (radial EBUS) consists of a 1.4-mm-diameter catheter with a 20 MHz ultrasound probe on the tip capable of being placed through the working channel of the bronchoscope into the lung periphery. Use of this device permits real-time confirmation that the probe is being extended into or adjacent to a lung nodule of interest to enhance biopsy yield (Figure 10.5). Use of a plastic outer sheath over the radial EBUS probe permits removal of the probe and insertion of sampling tools such as biopsy forceps to be guided to the same location.

A second technique known as electromagnetic navigational bronchoscopy (ENB) permits registration of a tracked device in the patient placed within an electromagnetic field with a recent CT scan of the chest during a bronchoscopic examination. This allows the operator to localize the tracked probe on the CT images, thereby aiding the selection of the correct bronchoscopic pathway to the peripheral lesion of interest. Use of radial EBUS and ENB equipment is often combined as the techniques provide complementary features in maximizing the localization of peripheral nodules. A recent metaanalysis examined the diagnostic yields achieved using the two methods and demonstrated that a diagnosis was obtained in 70 percent of patients investigated using either technique. Only one study was available that

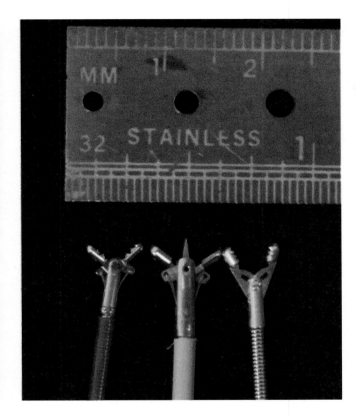

Figure 10.3 Three types of forceps available for use with the flexible bronchoscope. *Right to left:* small forceps with teeth; large, smooth-cupped forceps with center spike; and large forceps with teeth. The forceps fitted with a center spike are more commonly used for performing endobronchial biopsies.

reported on use of ENB and radial EBUS together and demonstrated diagnostic yields of 88 percent when the two approaches are combined 21.

After Procedure Care

Following bronchoscopy with TBB, patients should be observed in a recovery unit similar to other patients receiving conscious sedation. Given the increased risk of hemorrhage with TBB, we recommend that outpatients continue to not take their anticoagulants or antiplatelet agents until the morning following the procedure. Inpatients may resume anticoagulants such as heparin or enoxaparin 12 hours after the procedure.

Complications

Bronchoscopy with TBB is a safe procedure, and primary complications that arise with TBB are pneumothorax and hemorrhage. Pneumothorax occurs in 1–6 percent of patients undergoing TBB. Symptoms include chest pain, hemoptysis, and shortness of breath after the procedure. The need for chest radiography after TBB is controversial and is currently recommended only for patients who become symptomatic after the procedure. The use of fluoroscopy during TBB has not been shown to reduce risk of pneumothorax, although it is our practice to routinely use fluoroscopy during TBB and to perform a fluoroscopic screen for pneumothorax at the completion of the procedure.

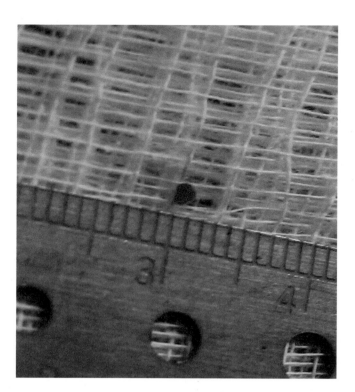

Figure 10.4 Representative TBB specimen. Note small size of tissue sample, approximately 1 mm in diameter.

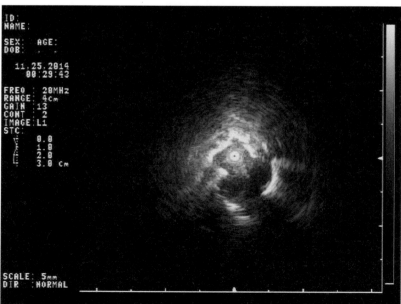

Figure 10.5 Endoscopic ultrasound image of a peripheral lung nodule showing aerated lung in the upper and left-hand side of the image with a small airway-centered pulmonary abnormality at the 3:00 to 6:00 o'clock position.

Significant hemorrhage, defined as >50 mL of blood, is observed in 2–9 percent of patients undergoing TBB. No randomized studies have been published on the optimal management of hemorrhage related to TBB, although several recommendations have been proposed by recognized experts. Zavala first described the wedge technique in 1976 whereby the tip of the bronchoscope is placed within the subsegment being biopsied using the technique described earlier. No data exist to suggest that the wedge technique decreases significant bleeding or related complications.

Additional therapeutic modalities that have been suggested include the use of iced saline administered via the working channel of the bronchoscope placed in the wedge position. Our practice is to give a 20-mL bolus of iced saline and withhold suctioning for several minutes to allow the cold fluid to induce local vasoconstriction. If the first bolus is unsuccessful, a second bolus is administered, repeating the observation period for several minutes, this may be followed by administration of 20 mL of 1:20,000 epinephrine if the bleeding continues. The patient should be placed with the hemorrhaging lung down to prevent soiling of the uninvolved lung. Using these measures, the majority of hemorrhages related to TBB will be controlled. Occasionally, the bleeding may be severe enough to require placement of an endobronchial blocker.

Conclusions

TBB is a useful and safe diagnostic tool for the appropriately trained pulmonologist. A wide variety of inflammatory, malignant, and infectious pulmonary diseases are amenable to diagnosis by TBB and, in the diagnosis of pulmonary malignancies, TBB is the procedure of choice in the appropriate setting. Complications are rare and generally easily managed by the well-trained physician.

Further Readings

Cazzadori A, DiPerri G, Todeschini G, et al. Transbronchial biopsy in the diagnosis of pulmonary infiltrates in immunocompromised patients. *Chest* 1995;107:101–106.

DuRand I, Blaikley J, Booton R, et al. British Thoracic Society guideline for diagnostic flexible bronchoscopy in adults. *Thorax* 2013;68:i1–i44.

Eberhardt R, Anantham D, Ernst A, Feller-Kopman D, Herth F. Multimodality bronchoscopic diagnosis of peripheral lung lesions: a randomized controlled trial. *Am J Respir Crit Care* 2007;176:36–41.

Ernst A, Eberhardt R, Wahidi M, Becker H, Herth F. Effect of routine clopidogrel use on bleeding complications after transbronchial biopsy in humans. *Chest* 2006;129:734–737.

Gilman M, Wang K. Transbronchial lung biopsy in sarcoidosis: an approach to determine the optimal number of biopsies. *Am Rev Respir Dis* 1980;122:721–724.

Glanville A. The role of bronchoscopic surveillance monitoring in the care of lung transplant recipients. *Semin Respir Crit Care Med* 2006;27:480–491.

Herth F, Becker H, Ernst A. Aspirin does not increase bleeding complications after transbronchial lung biopsy. *Chest* 2002;122:1461–1464.

Kearon C, Hirsh J. Management of anticoagulation before and after elective surgery. *N Engl J Med* 1997;336:1506–1511.

Leslie K, Gruden J, Parish J, Scholand M. Transbronchial biopsy interpretation in the patient with diffuse parenchymal lung disease. *Arch Pathol Lab Med* 2007;131:407–423.

Levy J, Spyropoulos A, Samama C, Douketis J. Direct oral anticoagulants new drugs and new concepts. *J Am Coll Cardiol Intv* 2014;7:1333–1351.

Matthay R, Farmer W, Odero D. Diagnostic fiberoptic bronchoscopy in the immunocompromised host with pulmonary infiltrates. *Thorax* 1977;32:539–545.

Naidich D, Sussman R, Kutcher W, Aranda C, Garay S, Ettenger N. Solitary pulmonary nodules. CT-bronchoscopic correlation. *Chest* 1988;93:595–598.

O'Donnell M, Kearon C, Johnson J, et al. Brief communication: preoperative anticoagulant activity after bridging low-molecular-weight heparin for temporary interruption of warfarin. *Ann Intern Med* 2007;146:184–187.

Papin T JL, Weg J. Transbronchial biopsy in the thrombocytopenic patient. *Chest* 1985;88:549–552.

Popovich J, Kvale P, Eichenhorn M, Radke J, Ohorodnik J, Fine G. Diagnostic accuracy of multiple biopsies from flexible fiberoptic bronchoscopy. A comparison of central versus peripheral carcinoma. *Am Rev Respir Dis* 1982;125:521–523.

Prakash U, Offord K, Stubbs S. Bronchoscopy in North America: the ACCP survey. *Chest* 1991;100:1668–1675.

Pue C, Pacht E. Complications of fiberoptic bronchoscopy at at university hospital. *Chest* 1995;107:430–432.

Schulman L, Smith C, Drusin R, Rose E, Enson Y, Reemtsma K. Utility of airway endoscopy in the diagnosis of respiratory complications of cardiac transplantation. *Chest* 1988;93:960–967.

Scott J, FRadet G, Smyth R, et al. Prospective study of transbronchial biopsies in the management of heart-lung and single lung transplant patients. *J Heart Lung Transplant* 1991;10:626–636.

Stover D, Zaman M, Hajdu S, Lange M, Gold J, Armstrong D. Bronchoalveolar lavage in the diagnosis of diffuse pulmonary infiltrates in the immunosuppressed host. *Ann Intern Med* 1984;101:1–7.

Wahidi M, Roca A, Hollingsworth J, Govert J, Feller-Kopman D, Ernst A. Contraindications and safety of transbronchial lung biopsy via flexible bronchoscopy. *Respiration* 2005;72:285–295.

Wang J, Nietert P, Silvestri G. Meta-analysis of guided bronchoscopy for the evaluation of the pulmonary nodule. *Chest* 2012;142:385–393.

Zavala D. Pulmonary hemorrhage in fiberoptic transbronchial biopsy. *Chest* 1976;70:585–588.

Transbronchial Needle Aspiration

William Fischer and David Feller-Kopman

Introduction

Transbronchial needle aspiration (TBNA) is a technique that has revolutionized the diagnosis of mediastinal pathology by enabling intrathoracic nodal sampling in a minimally invasive manner. The sampling of paratracheal masses using an esophageal varix needle passed through a rigid bronchoscope was initially described by Ko-Pen Wang in 1978. The following year Oho and colleagues created a needle that could be passed through a flexible bronchoscope, thus ushering in a novel modality for sampling intrathoracic lymph nodes without surgical intervention. Over the last 30 years, the technique of TBNA has been relatively unchanged, although the indications for TBNA have expanded to include sampling of hilar lymph nodes, submucosal disease, visible endobronchial lesions, as well as peripheral nodules. The recent development of advanced imaging such as computed tomography (CT) fluoroscopy, electromagnetic/virtual bronchoscopic navigation, and endobronchial ultrasound (EBUS) now allows real-time visualization of lymph node sampling. Because of these advances, TBNA has emerged as the first line of intrathoracic lymph node sampling for the diagnosis, staging, and prognosis of bronchogenic carcinoma, sarcoidosis, and even infectious diseases.

Bronchogenic carcinoma is the leading cause of cancer death in both men and women in the United States as well as in several other countries. Therapeutic options and prognoses are heavily dependent on accurate staging, and nodal staging is a key component of determining overall clinical stage (Figure 11.1). Non-invasive radiologic staging is suboptimal with sensitivities ranging from 51 to 74 percent. Additionally, because radiologic staging has been demonstrated to differ markedly from pathologic staging, the American Thoracic Society (ATS), European Respiratory Society (ERS), and European Society of Cardiothoracic Surgery all recommend that pathologic evaluation of the mediastinum be obtained in all patients prior to surgical resection of lung cancer. Mediastinoscopy has long been the gold standard for obtaining tissue, with sensitivities and specificities of 80–90 percent and 100 percent, respectively. Comparatively, the overall sensitivity of TBNA is 78 percent. Despite a high specificity (99 percent), TBNA is limited by a higher false-negative rate compared with that of mediastinoscopy (28 percent vs. 11 percent). The yield with TBNA has been associated with tumor cell type (small cell > non-small cell > lymphoma), lymph node size, and lymph node location. EBUS-TBNA has been shown to have a sensitivity and specificity of approximately 94 percent and 100 percent, respectively, and its yield may be independent of lymph node size and location. Nonetheless, if TBNA is nondiagnostic, surgical sampling is still recommended to rule out mediastinal nodal involvement. As a minimally invasive procedure, TBNA offers the significant benefit of fewer complications and has been demonstrated to preclude surgery in as many as 66 percent of patients.

Stage 0	TIS	
Stage Ia	T1, N0, M0	
Stage Ib	T2, N0, M0	
Stage IIa	T1, N1, M0	Surgical cure possible
Stage IIb	T2, N1, M0 T3, N0, M0	
Stage IIIa	T1-3, N2, M0 T3, N1, M0	
Stage IIIb	T4, any N, M0 any T, N3, M0	
Stage IV	any T, any N, M1	Chemotherapy +/- Radiation

Figure 11.1 Possible treatment options for patients with non-small cell lung cancer.

TBNA can also be used for peripheral parenchymal opacities. For peripheral lung cancer, TBNA has been shown to have a higher diagnostic yield than brushing or transbronchial biopsy. Peripheral TBNA is the exclusive diagnostic modality in up to 35 percent of cases, can obtain diagnostic tissue in up to 76 percent of cases, and significantly increases the yield when combined with other modalities used to sample peripheral opacities such as bronchoalveolar lavage (BAL), brushing, and/or transbronchial biopsy.

The major limitation of TBNA is that it remains an underused technique. Two recent surveys have found that only 12 percent of pulmonologists routinely used conventional TBNA in the evaluation of malignant disease, though EBUS is certainly increasing the overall use of TBNA. This likely results from fears of not obtaining adequate tissue, fears of causing damage to the bronchoscope, as well as inadequate training during fellowship. Among these reasons, lack of training is likely the foremost reason for the underuse of TBNA in clinical practice.

Anatomy

It is crucial that the bronchoscopist become an expert in airway anatomy, and there are several excellent chapters and texts to assist with this process. In addition to the upper airway and the segmental anatomy of the lungs, it is essential to have a comprehensive understanding of the anatomy external to the airway, primarily the intrathoracic vessels and lymph nodes. To maximize the sensitivity of TBNA, Wang proposed a staging system and anatomic guide for needle placement as defined by the CT scan and bronchoscopic imaging. Although extremely useful to the bronchoscopist, this lymph node map has one important limitation in that the nodal stations do not correspond exactly to those used by radiologists and thoracic surgeons. For example, in the system proposed by Wang, the left paratracheal station (4L) is also called the "aortic-pulmonary window." On the ATS/ERS lymph node map, however, the aortic-pulmonary window actually refers to station five and six nodes, which lie on the lateral side of the ligamentum arteriosum, and are therefore inaccessible by TBNA. As communication with our colleagues is essential, we recommend using the system proposed by the IASLC (Figure 11.2). That way, when the surgeons and radiologists refer to a left paratracheal lymph node (station 4L), everyone will be on the same page.

To improve one's yield, Wang suggested flipping the right and left CT images to help visualize the anatomic location of the lymph node relative to the airway during the procedure. Virtual bronchoscopy, by making the airway wall translucent and highlighting the target

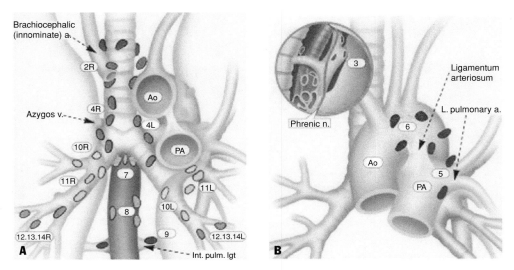

Figure 11.2 IASLC lymph node map (From: *J Thorac Oncol 2009;4:568.*)

lymph node, may also aid the bronchoscopist by having the visual of the relevant anatomy in the "mind's eye" during the procedure. The major drawback to these techniques is that the bronchoscopist is still required to mentally transpose the images during the procedure, and remains uncertain as to final needle position. Failure to place the needle directly into the lesion remains the leading cause of a lower yield on biopsy. Among lymph nodes of equivalent size, right paratracheal (4R) and subcarinal (7) stations have been shown to have a higher diagnostic yield than nodes in other stations. As such, these should be the first nodal stations attempted by novice operators.

Equipment

Although there are many different types of TBNA needles available for use, they can be divided into two broad categories: histology (19-gauge) and cytology (22-gauge) needles. Some histology needles have an inner 21-gauge needle and an outer 19-gauge needle, whereas others are a single 19-gauge needle. There has never been, and likely will never be, a study showing that one particular needle is better than another. Therefore, the bronchoscopist should familiarize him- or herself with one particular histology needle and one particular cytology needle.

Schenk and colleagues have shown that the 19-gauge needle provides a higher diagnostic yield as compared with that of the 22-gauge needle when used for lung cancer staging. All transbronchial needles consist of (1) a distal retractable sharp beveled needle, (2) a flexible catheter with a metal hub at the distal end, (3) a proximal control device used to manipulate the needle, and (4) a proximal side port through which suction can be applied.

Technique

When used for the staging of non-small cell lung cancer (NSCLC), it is of utmost importance to avoid false-positive results, which would have the clinical effect of upstaging a patient, and potentially precluding curative surgery. For this reason, TBNA should be the first procedure

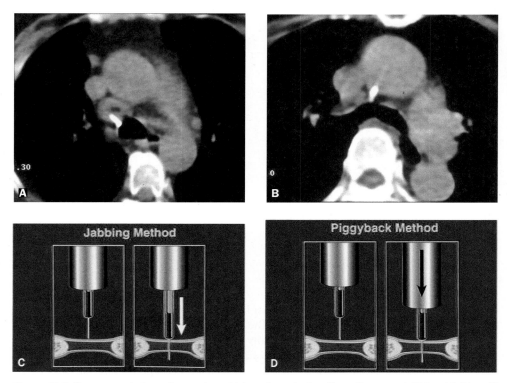

Figure 11.3 Common techniques for transbronchial needle aspiration. (From: Dasgupta A, Mehta AC, Wang KP. Transbronchial needle aspiration. *Semin Respir Crit Care Med.* 1997;18:571–581.)

performed during the bronchoscopy, and the lymph node station that would place the patient at the highest stage should be sampled first. For example, in the case of a patient with a T2 lesion in the left upper lobe, with adenopathy in stations 4L, 4R, and 7, the 4R node should be sampled first, as it would be considered N3, and therefore make the patient stage IIIb, and therefore not a surgical candidate. If the bronchoscopist attempted a BAL, brush, and transbronchial biopsy of the left upper lobe lesion first, the working channel of the bronchoscope could become contaminated and provide a false-positive result for subsequent TBNAs.

The Golden Rule of TBNA is "never advance the catheter in the bronchoscope with the needle out." A corollary to this rule is that the bronchoscopist is only as good as his or her support staff. It is essential to train your assistant prior to performing the procedure to be sure that he or she knows how to operate the needle. When the bronchoscope is in the desired location, the operator should keep the tip of the bronchoscope midline in the airway and advance the needle assembly through the working channel of the bronchoscope, making sure that the needle is retracted into the metal needle hub. After the catheter tip is visible within the bronchial lumen, the needle is advanced and locked into place. If at any time prior to needle insertion into the airway, the needle tip is *not* visible, it should immediately be retracted by the assistant. Once the bronchoscope is at the level of the target lymph node, the bronchoscope is flexed up so that the needle tip is as perpendicular to the airway wall as possible. Passage of the needle through the airway wall can occur in one of four methods, as described by Dasgupta and Mehta (Figure 11.3).

Jabbing Method

This method begins by retracting the catheter and extended needle so that only the tip of the needle is visible, again being careful not to withdraw the needle tip into the bronchoscope. The bronchoscope is flexed to position the needle perpendicular to the airway wall, and the needle is then advanced while the bronchoscope is held stationary.

Piggyback Method

As with the jabbing method, the extended needle is withdrawn such that only the tip of the needle is visible. Force is then applied to the bronchoscope and the needle–catheter apparatus until the needle penetrates the target lymph node. The bronchoscope thus provides a rigid support to the flexible needle to penetrate the bronchial wall.

Hub Against the Wall Method

This method begins with placement of the catheter hub against the airway wall adjacent to the target lymph node with the needle retracted in the hub. The needle is then deployed directly into the target tissue.

Cough Method

With the needle exposed through the catheter, it is positioned against the target lymph node. The patient is then instructed to cough, thereby pushing the bronchial wall against the needle.

In our practice, we typically start with the jabbing method; however, certain circumstances may require other techniques, and we will often use more than one method in any given procedure.

When in the target lesion, suction should be applied to ensure that the needle has not passed into a vessel. If blood is aspirated, suction should be released, the needle retracted, and another location selected. If blood is not aspirated, the needle should be passed in and out of the target. The syringe should then be disconnected from the catheter, the bronchoscope placed in a neutral position, and the needle withdrawn back into the catheter. The catheter is then removed in a single smooth motion from the bronchoscope.

Although one study suggests that, for NSCLC, there is diminishing return after seven passes at a given lymph node, a more recent study by Diacon's group suggests that this may occur after four needle passes. As stated earlier, factors such as underlying tumor histology, lymph node size, and station may influence these recommendations.

Specimen Processing and Interpretation

All material from the biopsy should be processed to maximize the yield from the procedure. A sample from a 19-gauge needle can be sent in formalin as a "core biopsy" to surgical pathology or be processed by cytopathology. Samples from a 22-gauge needle, however, should all be processed by cytopathology. It is important to talk to the surgical and cytopathology departments at one's institution to determine how they prefer their specimens. Some institutions have rapid on-site evaluation (ROSE) and may prefer that the specimen be placed directly on a glass slide for immediate staging, whereas other institutions prefer that the material for cytologic analysis be placed in CytoLyt or another medium. Several studies have shown that the use of ROSE is associated with a reduction in the number of inadequate specimens. This may be less of an issue with the development of real-time imaging provided by EBUS, but we still feel that it is important to review the results from all cases. This serves to enhance one's technique and provide feedback as to what worked and what did not for a particular needle pass. A major caveat for ROSE is the potential for a false-positive result that leads to premature termination of the procedure. As such, it is crucial that the cytopathologists be experienced in interpreting TBNA and only state that they have an adequate tissue sample when they are confident. Additionally, it is crucial to obtain enough tissue for analysis of genetic tumor markers, a diagnosis of "cancer," or even "adenocarcinoma" isn't adequate.

As TBNA does not have a 100 percent negative predictive value, we do prefer the term "nondiagnostic" to "negative." This is an important concept to explain to the patient as well, as, if the TBNA does not provide an answer, it may be essential to take the next step, perhaps a mediastinoscopy, and obtain more tissue.

Complications

TBNA is perhaps the safest bronchoscopic procedure available, with an overall complication rate of 0.26 percent. There have been case reports of bleeding, infection, pneumothorax, and pneumomediastinum; however, serious adverse effects are much less frequent when compared with those from transbronchial biopsy or surgical biopsy.

Improving the Yield

Clearly, experience counts. In a recent study by Hsu and colleagues, the sensitivity of TBNA increased from 33 to 81 percent over a period of 3.5 years. To gain experience, we recommend a commitment to learning mediastinal anatomy, understanding the technique from a conceptual standpoint, practicing the procedure on either a simulator or other model to gain the psychomotor skills, and then performing the procedure on as many patients with mediastinal and hilar adenopathy as possible. Feedback is essential, and it is crucial to review all cytology/pathology samples and to try to reference each pass with the technique used to obtain the tissue. This is a key benefit that ROSE can provide during the learning curve of TBNA.

The use of 19-gauge histology needles has been shown to increase the yield when compared with the use of cytology (22-gauge) needles, especially for nonmalignant disease. As earlier, we recommend that the operator become familiar with both a histology and a cytology needle. If the diagnosis leading the differential is not malignancy, the histology needle should be used.

The use of CT fluoroscopy (CTF) can be used to provide real-time confirmation of needle location. As opposed to standard fluoroscopy, which is typically used only in two dimensions, CT provides the ability to visualize the target in three dimensions and provides real-time three-dimensional confirmation of the appropriate (Figure 11.4A) and inappropriate (Figure 11.4B) biopsy sites. A study by Goldberg and colleagues analyzed data from 12 patients who underwent CTF-guided TBNA via a "quick-check" technique after having previously undergone non-diagnostic conventional BNA. A diagnosis was made in all patients, with a mean procedure time and number of aspirates similar to historical controls. Additionally, CTF confirmed that only six of the initial 18 (33 percent) needle passes were properly positioned within the target lymph node. With guidance, the rate of subsequent successful passes increased to 62 percent. Despite the fact that the TBNAs were performed by an experienced interventional pulmonologist, 42 percent of the needle insertions were not in the intended target. Six insertions (5.2 percent) were seen to have penetrated great vessels

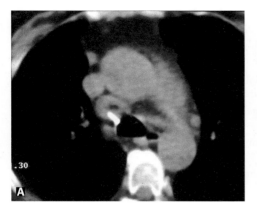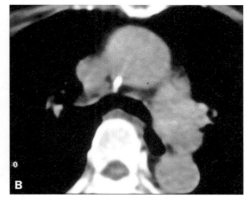

Figure 11.4 CTF showing **(A)** needle appropriately placed in station 4R node and **(B)** needle in aorta.

(four in the pulmonary artery, and one each in the left atrium and aorta); however, all of these were without complication.

Ernst's group went on to describe their results obtained by CTF in 32 patients with hilar and mediastinal adenopathy. As the yield with conventional TBNA is relatively high for nodes in the subcarinal and precarinal stations, patients with adenopathy in these areas were required to have a prior nondiagnostic TBNA to be included in the study. Adequate tissue was obtained in 28 patients (87.5 percent), and a specific diagnosis was made in 22 (68.8 percent). One patient had a false-negative CTF-guided TBNA. The authors conclude that, although CTF is not a substitute for good TBNA technique, it is an extremely helpful tool to improve the yield of TBNA in small and less accessible nodes.

EBUS is another important modality used to help improve accuracy of TBNA. Like CTF, EBUS has also been shown to significantly improve the yield of TBNA. Recently, a bronchoscope with a dedicated ultrasound probe and distinct working channel was developed (Olympus Corporation, Tokyo, Japan), and has the benefit of providing real-time guidance for TBNA of mediastinal and hilar lymph nodes, with excellent results. The sensitivity, specificity, and negative predictive value for EBUS-TBNA are 98.7, 100, and 97 percent, respectively. For lymphoma, EBUS-TBNA has been shown to have sensitivity, specificity, and negative predicative value of 91, 100, and 93 percent, respectively, despite the fact that the currently available needle for use in EBUS-TBNA is 22 gauge. Herth and colleagues have recently shown that, even in the presence of a radiographically normal mediastinum (as defined by no nodes > 1 cm on CT), EBUS identified malignancy in nearly 20 percent of patients, and avoided surgery in 17 percent. The use of EBUS has also been shown to improve subsequent yield when performing conventional TBNA.

Summary

Despite TBNA being available for nearly 30 years, it remains one of the most underused tools of the pulmonologist. TBNA is an extremely safe procedure and should be routinely used to sample mediastinal and hilar lymph nodes, endobronchial lesions, as well as parenchymal opacities. EBUS-TBNA now allows real-time guidance of lymph nodes and may preclude the need for surgery in a significant number of patients. These new technologies, however, do not make one a better bronchoscopist; we therefore recommend dedicated training and continued practice.

Further Readings

American Thoracic Society and The European Respiratory Society. Pretreatment evaluation of non-small-cell lung cancer. *Am J Respir Crit Care Med*. 1997;156(1):320–332.

Becker HD. *Atlas of Bronchoscopy: Technique, Diagnosis, Differential Diagnosis, Therapy*. Philadelphia: BC Decker; 1991.

Cordovilla R, Torracci AM, Garcia-Macias MC. Enhancement of conventional TBNA outcome after EBUS training. *J Bronchology Interv Pulmonol*. 2014;21:322–326.

Cortese DA, Prakash UBS. Anatomy for the bronchoscopist. In: Prakash UBS, ed. *Bronchoscopy*. New York: Raven Press, Ltd.; 1994:13–42.

Dasgupta A, Mehta AC. Transbronchial needle aspiration. An underused diagnostic technique. *Clin Chest Med*. 1999;20(1):39–51.

Dasgupta A, Mehta A, Wang KP. Transbronchial needle aspiration. *Semin Respir Crit Care Med*. 1997; 18:571–581.

Davenport RD. Rapid on-site evaluation of transbronchial aspirates. *Chest*. 1990;98(1):59–61.

De Leyn P, Lardinois D, Van Schil PE, Rami-Porta R, Passlick B, Zielinski M, Waller DA, Lerut T, Weder W. ESTS guidelines for preoperative lymph node staging for non-small cell lung cancer. *Eur J Cardiothorac Surg*. 2007;32(1):1–8.

Detterbeck FC, Jantz MA, Wallace M, Vansteenkiste J, Silvestri G. Invasive mediastinal staging of lung cancer: ACCP evidence-based clinical practice guidelines (2nd ed.). *Chest*. 2007;132(3 Suppl): 202S–220S.

Diacon AH, Schuurmans MM, Theron J, Brundyn K, Louw M, Wright CA, Bolliger CT. Transbronchial needle aspirates: how many passes per target site? *Eur Respir J*. 2007;29(1):112–116.

Diette GB, White P Jr, Terry P, Jenckes M, Rosenthal D, Rubin HR. Utility of on-site cytopathology assessment for bronchoscopic evaluation of lung masses and adenopathy. *Chest*. 2000;117(4): 1186–1190.

Ernst A, Feller-Kopman D, Herth FJ. Endobronchial ultrasound in the diagnosis and staging of lung cancer and other thoracic tumors. *Semin Thorac Cardiovasc Surg*. 2007;19(3):201–205.

Feller-Kopman DJ, Brigham E, Lechtzin N, Gilbert C, Akulian J, Yarmus L. Training perspective: the impact of starting an endobronchial ultrasound program at a major academic center on fellow's training of transbronchial needle aspiration. *Ann Am Thorac Soc*. 2013;10:127–130.

Garpestad E, Goldberg SN, Herth F, Garland R, LoCicero J, Thurer R, Ernst A. CT fluoroscopy guidance for transbronchial needle aspiration: an experience in 35 patients. *Chest*. 2001;119(2): 329–332.

Goldberg SN, Raptopoulos V, Boiselle PM, Edinburgh KJ, Ernst A. Mediastinal lymphadenopathy: diagnostic yield of transbronchial mediastinal lymph node biopsy with CT fluoroscopic guidance – initial experience. *Radiology*. 2000;216(3):764–767.

Haponik EF, Shure D. Underutilization of transbronchial needle aspiration: experiences of current pulmonary fellows. *Chest*. 1997;112(1):251–253.

Harrow EM, Abi-Saleh W, Blum J, Harkin T, Gasparini S, Addrizzo-Harris DJ, Arroliga AC, Wight G, Mehta AC. The utility of transbronchial needle aspiration in the staging of bronchogenic carcinoma. *Am J Respir Crit Care Med*. 2000;161(2 Pt 1):601–607.

Herth F, Becker HD, Ernst A. Conventional vs endobronchial ultrasound-guided transbronchial needle aspiration: a randomized trial. *Chest*. 2004;125(1):322–325.

Herth FJ, Becker HD, Ernst A. Ultrasound-guided transbronchial needle aspiration: an experience in 242 patients. *Chest*. 2003;123(2):604–607.

Herth FJ, Eberhardt R, Vilmann P, Krasnik M, Ernst A. Real-time, endobronchial ultrasound-guided, transbronchial needle aspiration: a new method for sampling mediastinal lymph nodes. *Thorax*. 2006;61(9): 795–798. Epub May 31, 2006.

Herth FJF, Ernst A, Eberhardt R, Vilmann P, Dienemann H, Krasnik M. Endobronchial ultrasound-guided transbronchial needle aspiration of lymph nodes in the radiologically normal mediastinum. *Eur Respir J*. 2006;28(5):910–914.

Holty JE, Kuschner WG, Gould MK. Accuracy of transbronchial needle aspiration for mediastinal staging of non-small cell lung cancer: a meta-analysis. *Thorax*. 2005;60(11):949–955.

Hsu LH, Liu CC, Ko JS. Education and experience improve the performance of transbronchial needle aspiration: a learning curve at a cancer center. *Chest*. 2004;125(2):532–540.

Kennedy MP, Jimenez CA, Bruzzi JF, Mhatre AD, Lei X, Giles FJ, Fanning T, Morice RC, Eapen GA. Endobronchial ultrasound guided transbronchial needle aspiration in the diagnosis of lymphoma. *Thorax*. 2008;63(4):360–365.

Oho K, Kato H, Ogawa I, Hayashi N, Hayata Y. A new needle for transfiberoptic bronchoscopic use. *Chest*. 1979;76(4):492.

Patel NM, Pohlman A, Husain A, Noth I, Hall JB, Kress JP. Conventional transbronchial needle aspiration decreases the rate of surgical sampling of intrathoracic lymphadenopathy. *Chest*. 2007; 131(3):773–778.

Rusch V, Asamura H, Watanabe H, Giroux DJ, Rami-Porta R, Goldstraw P. The IASLC Lung Cancer Staging Project. A proposal for a new international lymph node map in the forthcoming seventh edition of the TNM Classification of Lung Cancer. *J Thorac Oncol*. 2009;4:568–577.

Schenk DA, Chambers SL, Derdak S, Komadina KH, Pickard JS, Strollo PJ, Lewis RE, Patefield AJ, Henderson JH. Comparison of the Wang 19-gauge and 22-gauge needles in the mediastinal staging of lung cancer. *Am Rev Respir Dis*. 1993;147(5):1251–1258.

Shure D, Fedullo PF. Transbronchial needle aspiration of peripheral masses. *Am Rev Respir Dis*. 1983; 128(6):1090–1092.

Silvestri GA, Gould MK, Margolis ML, Tanoue LT, McCrory D, Toloza E, Detterbeck F. Noninvasive staging of non-small cell lung cancer: ACCP evidenced-based clinical practice guidelines (2nd ed.). *Chest*. 2007;132(3 Suppl):178S–201S.

Vincent BD, El-Bayoumi E, Hoffman B, Doelken P, DeRosimo J, Reed C, Silvestri GA. Real-time endobronchial ultrasound-guided transbronchial lymph node aspiration. *Ann Thorac Surg*. 2008; 85(1):224–230.

Wang KP. Staging of bronchogenic carcinoma by bronchoscopy. *Chest*. 1994;106(2):588–593.

Wang KP, Terry P, Marsh B. Bronchoscopic needle aspiration biopsy of paratracheal tumors. *Am Rev Respir Dis*. 1978;118(1):17–21.

Yasufuku K, Chiyo M, Sekine Y, Chhajed PN, Shibuya K, Iizasa T, Fujisawa T. Real-time endobronchial ultrasound-guided transbronchial needle aspiration of mediastinal and hilar lymph nodes. *Chest*. 2004;126(1):122–128.

Chapter 12

Bronchoscopy in the Intensive Care Unit

Jed A. Gorden

In the future, as at present, the internist will tap and look and listen on the outside of the chest … ; the roentgenologist will continue to look through the patient; but in a continually increasing proportion of cases, the surgeon, the internist and the roentgenologist will ask the bronchoscopist to look inside the patient.
Chevalier Jackson, MD 1928

Introduction

Bronchoscopy is an essential tool in critical care medicine and an increasingly ubiquitous presence in the hospital. The ease, safety, and portability of bronchoscopy make it one of the most commonly requested invasive procedures in the ICU setting.

The ready access of bronchoscopy to intensivists has broadened the pulmonary diagnostic and therapeutic capabilities in critically ill patients, but like many technologies it also raises certain challenges in its appropriate application. Technology is not a substitute for good clinical judgment; operators must assess patient safety and perform procedures with attention to patient comfort with knowledge of potential complications and a management plan for complications including respiratory failure, pneumothorax, etc.

In this chapter I hope to outline the most common consultations and appropriate uses for bronchoscopy in the ICU. The overwhelming number of indications will be for diagnostic questions, all though some therapeutic indications exist. Common indications for bronchoscopy in the ICU are listed in Table 12.1.

Route of Bronchoscopy in the ICU

Bronchoscopy performed in the ICU on critically ill patients is safe, but an appropriate risk benefit analysis is always necessary. Bronchoscopy can be performed on both intubated and extubated patients but when performing bronchoscopy on extubated patients stability of oxygenation and ventilation must be assessed and the risk of respiratory failure either from sedation medications or the procedure itself must be evaluated.

Bronchoscopy in the Extubated Patient

Bronchoscopy on the extubated patient can be performed either via the oral route using a bite block or transnasaly. The patient must have oxygen requirements that can be managed by reasonable supplementation and cannot have impending respiratory failure or requirements for noninvasive ventilation like CPAP or BIPAP. The patient should have a mental status that permits the use of sedation and analgesia. The bronchoscopist when performing

Table 12.1 Indications for Bronchoscopy in the ICU

Diagnostic	Therapeutic
Secretion/atelectasis management	Hemoptysis
Fever/Ventilator associated Pneumonia	Foreign body removal
Hemoptysis	Difficult intubations
Failed extubation	Percutaneous traceostomy guidance
Undiagnosed X-ray change/	
Central airway obstruction	

bronchoscopy on an extubated ICU patient must be skilled in intubation either by direct laryngoscopy or over a bronchoscope, in case of respiratory failure. Contraindications to flexible bronchoscopy without intubation include: (1) Respiratory rate > 30 bpm, (2) Clinical use of accessory muscles signifying impending respiratory failure, (3) $PaO^2 < 70$ mm Hg or $SaO^2 < 90$ percent with supplemental oxygen, (4) Requirement for minimally invasive BiCAP/CPAP ventilation, (5) Significantly altered mental status.

Bronchoscopy in the Intubated Patient

Performing bronchoscopy through an endotracheal tube (ETT) in the ICU is a common procedure. The endotracheal tube should be placed prior to the procedure if the patient's respiratory status is felt to be fragile and the information from bronchoscopy is critical to patient care. The most common sizes for endotracheal tubes in adults are: 7.0 mm, 7.5 mm, and 8.0 mm. Bronchoscopes are commonly referred to as "diagnostic" and "therapeutic" based on the size of the suction channel and the overall size of the bronchoscope. Therapeutic bronchoscopes are larger and typically have a suction channel ≥2.8 mm, they are best suited to viscous and larger volume airway secretions. Diagnostic scopes are smaller with working channels ≤2.8 mm. The bronchoscope must easily pass through the inner lumen of the ETT and permit exhaled gas to escape to prevent air trapping, Table 12.2 shows common ETT

Table 12.2 Endotracheal Tube (ETT) Size Correlation with Bronchoscope Size

Sizes of Scopes				
Internal diameter of endotracheal or tracheotomy tube at least 2 mm larger than bronchoscope diameter				
Bronchoscope Models	Inner Diameter of suction port	Outer Diameter of distal end of Bronchoscope	ENDTRACHEAL TUBES Sizes related to scope model size	TRACHEOSTOMY TUBES Sizes related to scope model size
BF-XP160F	1.2 mm	2.8 mm	ETT 5.0 <	PORTEX # 6 / 5 MM ID
BF-3C160	1.2 mm	3.8 mm	ETT 6.0 <	PORTEX # 7 / 6 MM ID
BF-P180	2.0 mm	4.9 mm	ETT 7.0 <	PORTEX # 8 / 7 MM ID
BF-Q180	2.0 mm	5.1 mm	ETT 7.0 <	PORTEX # 9 / 8 MM ID
BF-1T180	3.0 mm	6.0 mm	ETT 8.0 <	PORTEX # 10 / 9 MM ID
BF-XT160	3.2 mm	6.3 mm	ETT 9.0 <	

Will not fit with tower interface and light source.

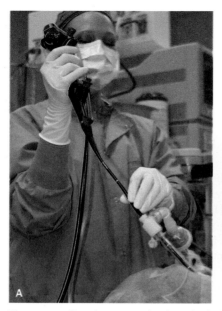
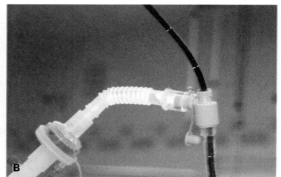

Figure 12.1 Bronchoscope and endotracheal tube adapter.

sizes and size appropriate bronchoscopes. If the patient has a smaller-diameter ETT limiting bronchoscopy, the intensivist should consider changing the ETT to a larger diameter. Remember a smaller bronchoscope will have a smaller working channel and considerably less suctioning capability limiting visibility and decreasing suctioning of secretions and specimen acquisition. When performing bronchoscopy on the mechanically ventilated patient an adapter is required on the end of the endotracheal tube to ensure that tidal volume and PEEP are maintained during the procedure (Figure 12.1).

Sedation

When performing bronchoscopy on either the intubated or extubated patient in the intensive care unit sedation is required. Typical sedation involves the use of an analgesic and a sedative, the most common combination is opiates and benzodiazepines but sedation can be individualized to your specific ICU protocol. Topical sedation for both the intubated and extubated patient cannot be overlooked. In the extubated patient topical anesthesia in the posterior pharynx and airway limits the gag reflex. In the intubated patient topical anesthesia down the ETT or tracheostomy tube minimizes airway irritation and cough. When bronchoscopy is to be performed via the nasal route the nares must be adequately anaesthetized with topical gels. For ICU bronchoscopy routine neuromuscular blockade is not required.

In general patients who are not and will not need to be intubated and require bronchoscopy in the ICU should have had no oral or tube feed intake (NPO) for six hours prior to the procedure. NPO status is required to minimize the risk of aspiration and further compromise to critically ill patients; this is less of a concern in patients who already have an endotracheal tube in place. The patient can be maintained with intravenous hydration during this period.

Box 12.1 Contraindications to Bronchoscopy in the ICU

- Patient PaO^2 < 60–80 mm Hg on 100% FiO^2
- Acute ischemic heart disease (MI) or unstable angina
- Hypotension with systemic blood pressure < 90 mm Hg
- Critical cardiac dysrhythmias
- Known increased intracranial pressures

Bronchoscopy Safety Checklist

- Continuous oxygen saturation monitoring
- Hemodynamic monitoring cycled every 2–5 minutes
- Continuous cardiac rate and rhythm monitoring
- Ventilated patients increase FiO^2 to 100 percent 5–15 minutes prior to procedure
- Nursing support for sedation and monitoring
- Respiratory therapy support for ventilator management monitoring of minute ventilation and pressure limited volume loss
- Technical support to assist with procedure lavage, etc.

Safety of Bronchoscopy in the Critically Ill

Flexible bronchoscopy and sample acquisition from the airways is a valuable tool of the critical care physician. Bronchoscopy is considered safe in critically ill patients with both respiratory failure and hemodynamic impairment as long as simple principles are followed. Steinberg and colleagues prospectively studied the effects of bronchoscopy with bronchoalveolar lavage (BAL) or protected brush specimen (PSB) on 110 patients who met clinical criteria for adult respiratory distress syndrome (ARDS). In their study there was no statistically significant change in the patients mean PaO^2/FIO^2 ratio, mean arterial pressure (MAP), or heart rate (HR) when comparing pre-procedure values to one-hour post procedure data. Approximately 5 percent of patients experienced oxygen desaturation to <90 percent none lasted longer than 15 minutes. No patients experienced prolonged effects from the transient desaturations or the procedure itself. Papazian et al focused on a group of 12 critically ill hemodynamically unstable patients who underwent bronchoscopy with BAL and PSB on inotropic or vasoactive support. No significant hemodynamic or ventilatory interventions were required during or after the procedures.

In all the studies demonstrating safety of bronchoscopy and BAL in critically ill patients safety was maintained despite the installation of 100–200 mL of 0.9 percent saline for lavage.

To safely perform bronchoscopy in critically ill patients a knowledgeable team is required. Staffing should include a respiratory therapist at the bedside for intubated and nonintubated patients, as well as a nurse present to assist with sedation and patient monitoring. The team must be familiar with bronchoscopy equipment set up, specimen acquisition, and ventilator management if relevant. A safety pause should be initiated prior to starting the procedure to insure the appropriate patient and procedure are identified and that all team members are present and focused on their responsibility. A safety checklist with indications and contraindications is outlined in Box 12.1. Bronchoscopy is relatively contraindicated in the following clinical circumstances until the acute clinical situation has stabilized: (1) PaO^2 <60–80 on 100 percent FiO^2, (2) acute ischemic heart disease or unstable angina, (3) hypotension

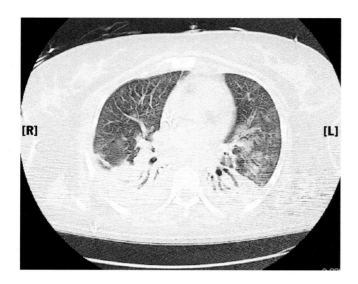

Figure 12.2 CT scan of patient with ARDS and airbronchograms and posterior lung consolidation.

[R]   [L]

with systolic blood pressure less than 90 mm Hg, (4) critical cardiac dysrhythmias, and (5) known increased intracranial pressure.

To safely perform bronchoscopy on critically ill patients the following is required: (1) continuous oxygen saturation monitoring, (2) monitoring of hemodynamics every 2–5 minutes, (3) In ventilated patients the FiO^2 should be increased to 100 percent 5–15 minutes prior to the procedure, (4) monitoring for loss of minute ventilation and pressure limited volume loss due to the presence of the bronchoscope in the airway increasing peak airway pressures.

Therapeutic Aspiration of Secretions

One of the most common consultations for bronchoscopy in the ICU is the management of retained secretions and atelectasis. In published series from the Mayo clinic ICU from 1985 to 1988 clearance of retained secretions accounted for 50 percent of ICU bronchoscopies and in a series from the University of California Davis from 1979 to 1980 63 percent of bronchoscopies were performed for this purpose. The use of bronchoscopy for retained secretions and atelectasis is the subject of strong convictions and little data. There is little doubt that bronchoscopy for therapeutic removal of secretions and aggressive pulmonary toilet is safe but its efficacy and impact on clinical outcomes remains unresolved. In 1979 Marini et al randomized 31 patients with acute lobar atelectasis to bronchoscopy followed by chest physiotherapy for 48 hours vs. chest physiotherapy alone for the same period without bronchoscopy; there was no clinically significant difference in outcomes of the two groups. In both groups the presence of air bronchograms (Figure 12.2) resulted in delayed recovery.

Bronchoscopy and BAL should not be considered first line therapy for routine pulmonary toilet and secretion clearance in the ICU. Bronchoscopy should be considered in cases of acute lobar collapse particularly with alterations in oxygenation status if routine suctioning fails (Figure 12.3). Patients who have undergone thoracic surgery with airway manipulation are an unstudied population but may benefit from bronchoscopic therapeutic aspiration of secretions due to airway edema or airway tortuosity complicating pulmonary toilet. The viscosity of secretions is important to consider inspissated secretions which often occlude

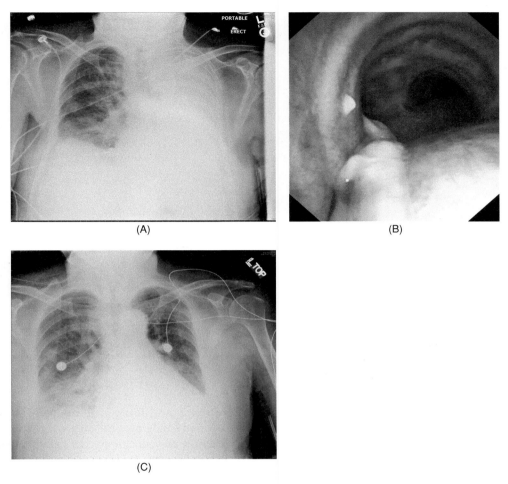

Figure 12.3 (A) Chest X-ray with occlusion from mucous plug **(B)** Endoluminal view of mucous plug **(C)** Chest X-ray with lung expansion following therapeutic aspiration of mucous plug

airway stents may be challenging to remove at the bedside and require more advanced endoscopic intervention (Figure 12.4).

Bronchoscopy; Febrile Neutropenia

Febrile neutropenic patients and patients with general immune compromise are a specialty group of patients often admitted to the ICU setting. Febrile neutropenia is considered an oncologic emergency and is most commonly associated with the use of chemotherapy or hematopoietic stem cell transplantation. The differential diagnosis for febrile neutropenia and pulmonary infiltrates can be broad with infection, bacterial, fungal, or viral being the most sinister. Other diagnoses include but are not limited to diffuse alveolar hemorrhage, radiation pneumonitis, drug induced toxicity, or malignancy itself.

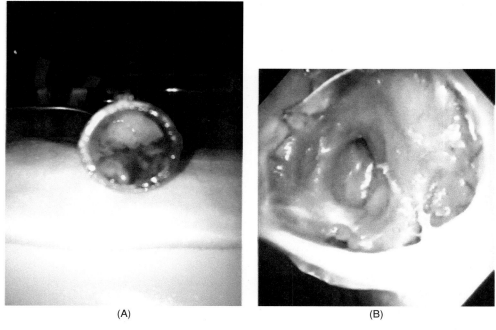

(A) (B)

Figure 12.4 **(A)** Silicone Y-stent with mucous impaction **(B)** Self expanding bronchial stent with inspissated secretions

Early use of empiric antibiotic therapy is the standard of care for this patient population, but flexible bronchoscopy is both safe and commonly used to augment the diagnostic work up. Diagnostic yield of flexible bronchoscopy in the febrile neutropenic patient in multiple studies has been shown to be approximately 50 percent. In a prospective series of neutropenic ICU patients the diagnostic yield of flexible bronchoscopy and BAL differed by cause of neutropenia. In patients who suffered febrile neutropenia as a result of high dose chemotherapy the diagnostic yield of bronchoscopy and BAL was 63 percent if the cause of neutropenia was stem cell transplantation the diagnostic yield fell to 38–47 percent.

Bronchoscopy in the febrile neutropenic patient in the ICU is safe with complications usually being minor and most always mirroring those of the general critically ill population. A unique clinical finding in this patient population in addition to their critical illness is often thrombocytopenia either as a result of medications or underlying illness. Bronchoscopy with BAL is safe in thrombocytopenic immune compromised patients with few reported incidences of life threatening epistaxis, hemoptysis, or alveolar hemorrhage.

Nearly all patients with febrile neutropenia are on empiric broad-spectrum antibiotics and bronchoscopy should not delay empiric antibiotic coverage. Published series report a change in antimicrobial therapy based on BAL results in 28–51 percent of the time. Viral and fungal disease often account for most therapeutic changes. A non-diagnostic bronchoscopy with BAL is insufficient to discontinue antimicrobial therapy in this patient population. Trans bronchial biopsy in the febrile neutropenic patient adds little to the diagnostic yield and is usually considered contraindicated in the setting of thrombocytopenia.

It is imperative that bronchoscopists coordinate with relevant infectious disease to insure all appropriate samples are sent to avoid the need for repeat procedures.

Ventilator-Associated Pneumonia

Ventilator-associated pneumonia (VAP) is a common and serious problem facing critically ill patients on mechanical ventilation. The diagnosis of VAP is made when a patient who has been on mechanical ventilation for ≥ 48 hours develops a new or progressive pulmonary infiltrate on X-ray and positive respiratory culture specimens. It is estimated that 8–28 percent of intubated patients requiring mechanical ventilation will develop a ventilator-associated pneumonia. Mortality associated with VAP is high between 24 and 50 percent. Given the severe consequences associated with VAP it is critical that a timely and accurate diagnosis is made. Bronchoscopy is an excellent tool for obtaining microbiology specimens, either bronchoalveolar lavage (BAL) or protected specimen brush (PSB), from focal affected areas identified on CXR in patients with suspected VAP. Quantitative cultures from BAL or PSB specimens help to tailor antibiotic selection and have been associated with decreased antibiotic usage but the impact of bronchoscopy in VAP on mortality remains controversial. Bronchoscopy should not delay antimicrobial therapy particularly in ICU cultures where 24-hour bronchoscopy services are not available.

Hemoptysis

The goals in managing massive hemoptysis are securing the airway, identification of the bleeding source, isolation of the bleeding area to prevent soiling of the unaffected lung, and cessation of bleeding. No consensus definition exists for massive hemoptysis, the literature often quotes 100–600 mL/24 hours but it is most important to understand that problems come not from blood loss but impairment in gas exchange. Four hundred milliliters of blood in the alveolar space can significantly impair gas exchange with only a minor perturbation in vital signs. Bronchoscopy and radiology imaging are potent tools in identifying the cause and location of hemoptysis. Bronchoscopy allows for direct examination of the central airways for tumors or other bleeding diathesis as well as examination of segmental orifices to reveal the potential regional source of bleeding or at a minimum lateralize the source of bleeding to the left or right lung. Timing is crucial in localizing bleeding in cases of hemoptysis. Bronchoscopy when performed early either during active bleeding or within 24–48 hours can localize the bleeding 75–85 percent of the time, if bronchoscopy is delayed greater than 48 hours localization of bleeding drops to 25–50 percent.

Computed tomography imaging is far superior to conventional chest X-ray and greatly helps the bronchoscopist by creating a potential road map of airway and parynchymal abnormalities. The intensivist must take into account the patient's stability when considering the role of medical imaging because it would be inappropriate to transfer an unstable patient to radiology.

Localization of non-life threatening hemoptysis is best done employing the flexible bronchoscope. It is rapidly available, does not require general anesthesia, can be performed at the bedside, and allows for the most thorough airway survey. This rapid diagnostic survey helps with therapeutic planning. The primary limitations of flexible bronchoscopy are diminished visibility even in the presence of small volumes of blood and low suction capability. In the presence of active bleeding, it may be very difficult for the flexible bronchoscope to adequately

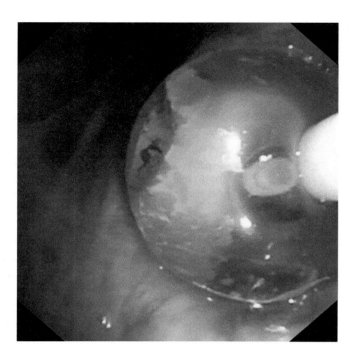

Figure 12.5 Endobronchial blocker.

obtain and maintain a clear airway, limiting both the goal of airway control, and the goal of bleeding localization.

Once the bleeding source has been localized good communication is required between the bronchoscopist and their therapeutic colleagues in interventional pulmonology, thoracic surgery, or interventional radiology. A number of interventional options are available for central airway bleeding lesions, beyond the scope of this review including heat energy sources; APC, laser, and cautery freezing delivery sources like cryotherapy are less effective in establishing hemostasis in airway bleeding. If the source of bleeding has been localized beyond the central airways good anatomical communication with interventional radiology colleagues is necessary for potential embolization procedures. In patients with known malignancy and central airway tumors consultation with interventional pulmonology colleagues or thoracic surgery for local control efforts followed by radiation oncology for more durable bleeding control.

If bleeding is extensive the use of endobronchial blockers is an important temporizing tool while awaiting more definitive therapy. Endobronchial blockers can be placed under direct vision using flexible bronchoscopy (Figure 12.5), once the blocker is inflated it should be deflated and the airway inspected at least every 24 hours.

In extreme life threatening cases selective intubation of either the right or left mainstem bronchi is required to prevent soiling the unaffected lung. This is best and most rapidly achieved by placing the endotracheal tube over the bronchoscope advancing the bronchoscope into the non-bleeding mainstem bronchus and advancing the endotracheal tube into the selected mainstem airway using the bronchoscope as a guide wire, inflate the balloon on the endotracheal tube to prevent soiling of the non-bleeding lung while awaiting definitive treatment.

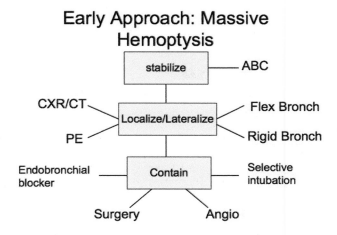

Figure 12.6 Algorithm for management of hemoptysis.

A practical approach to massive hemoptysis is outlined in Figure 12.6 but the principles include: (1) Early patient stabilization with attention to the airway and breathing and the potential need for intubation. (2) Early localization of bleeding with bronchoscopy and possible CT imaging. (3) Finally containment of bleeding with localized therapy or interventional radiology embolization.

Massive hemoptysis requires a true multidisciplinary approach and good early communication between intensivists and interventionalists from many disciplines including interventional pulmonology, thoracic surgery, interventional radiology, and radiation oncology.

Removal of Foreign Body

In March of 1897 Professor Killian was presented with a 63-year-old farmer with profound dyspnea, cough, and hemoptysis. Killian employing the Kirstein laryngoscope identified an object in the right main stem bronchus. Using cocaine anesthesia and the Muckulicz-Rosenhiem esophagoscope, Killian deployed graspers through the lumen of the scope to secure what turned out to be a pork bone fragment. The 8-mm diameter of the esophagoscope forced the en masse removal of the object and the scope, and thus the first documented bronchoscopic procedure was performed for a foreign body extraction.

Aspiration of a foreign body can lead to critical airway obstruction and respiratory distress or obstruction at the segmental level resulting in lobar collapse or a post obstructive pneumonia. The ease of access to the airways with bronchoscopy has had a dramatic impact on the sub acute and chronic sequela associated with airway foreign bodies. These are namely: respiratory distress, obstructive pneumonia, and lung abscess. The nature of aspirated foreign bodies has certain geographic and cultural variability. The most cited foreign body aspirations are vegetable matter, peanuts, or bones. Not all foreign bodies are aspirated out of hospital. Hospital appliances can find their way into the airway with particular attention to tracheal appliances including tracheal buttons. The most common adult age groups for foreign body aspiration are in the sixth and seventh decades of life. The predominance of aspirated foreign bodies occurs in children.

Flexible bronchoscopy is a powerful tool in the removal of aspirated foreign bodies; its safety and portability profile make it an excellent ICU bedside tool for this purpose. In one

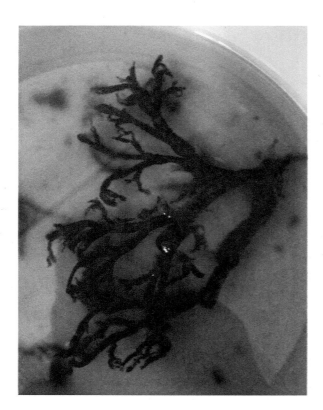

Figure 12.7 Clot and fibrin airway obstructing cast.

published series flexible bronchoscopy was successful in extracting the foreign body from the airway in 60 percent of cases. There are a number of tools specifically designed for the flexible bronchoscope including graspers and baskets for airway foreign body retrieval. When attempting to remove a foreign body from the airway a "therapeutic" bronchoscope with the larger working channel should be used. It is reasonable to initially attempt foreign body extraction with the flexible bronchoscope, with a high likelihood of success, but rigid bronchoscopy is a useful adjunct and prompt conversion to rigid bronchoscopy may save the patient from multiple interventions but requires transfer to the operating room.

It is generally thought that when aspiration occurs objects preferentially obstruct the right bronchial tree due to the anatomy and angle of entry into the right and left main stem bronchi off the trachea. In adults the left main stem bronchus branches at a more obtuse angle relative to the midline trachea in contrast to the right mainstem bronchus which maintains a more direct linear path with the trachea resulting in more frequent right mainstem bronchial intubations as well as aspiration of foreign objects. Hemorrhage into the tracheal bronchial tree can cause obstruction sometimes creating an airway cast (Figure 12.7).

Factors that can impact aspiration risk include; level of consciousness, age, and facial trauma when these factors are present coupled with unexplained lobar collapse with volume loss on chest X-ray or unexplained wheezing a diagnostic bronchoscopy should be considered to rule out an aspirated foreign body.

Bronchoscopy in Trauma

Airway trauma can occur as a result of external blunt force injuries or internal insults like the endotracheal tube stilet. Airway injuries can be readily identified by bedside ICU bronchoscopy. Common signs associated with tracheal or bronchial disruption include: pneumomediastinum post blunt trauma to the chest, persistent pneumothorax despite adequate chest tube evacuation in the setting of thoracic trauma, fracture of one or more of the first three ribs, and persistent pneumothorax and air leak in the early period post lung transplant suggesting anastamotic disruption.

In cases of persistent pneumomediastinum without other explanation airway injury can be suspected including airway injury sustained as a result of intubation with stilet or tracheostomy tube insertion. Typically this results in injury to the posterior membranous trachea or the right mainstem bronchus if the ETT is advanced too far. Again this can be readily diagnosed by diagnostic bronchoscopy but may require deflation of the balloon on the ETT and gentle withdrawal of the tube if the ETT has been advanced over the injury site.

Inhalation injury either steam or caustic substances warrants an airway inspection to access for airway sloughing and web stenosis formation. It can also be used to assess for laryngeal swelling and the need for securing a stable airway.

Failed Extubation

Failure to be able to liberate a patient from mechanical ventilation is a common problem in the ICU and most often reflects persistent critical illness and respiratory failure. In certain circumstances failure to extubate reflects a mechanical problem that increases the work of breathing. Specific mechanical problems that can be readily diagnosed by bronchoscopy are: Increased airway granulation tissue resulting in airway obstruction, tracheal stenosis, and tracheal bronchial malacia. Another unique circumstance is patients with tracheostomy tubes who have respiratory distress when the tracheostomy tube is caped or a passy meur valve is placed. This may represent the buildup of granulation tissue at the distal end of the tracheostomy tube or in the subglottic space. This is easily diagnosed by bedside bronchoscopy. Intubation injury can be subglottic creating a flap injury. The dissected flap can occlude the airway, often on exhalation when the endotracheal tube is removed, and result in post extubation stridor or post extubation respiratory failure (Figure 12.8).

ICU Difficult Airway Intubation

The bronchoscope should always be considered part of the difficult intubation armamentarium. When confronted with a difficult airway or patient with an unstable neck, intubation can be facilitated by placement of the endotracheal tube over the bronchoscope and then using the bronchoscopic optics to find the cords and pass into the trachea then advance the ETT over the bronchoscope into the airway. The larger the diameter scope, the easier it is to maneuver and to aspirate secretions to improve visibility. If smaller ETT are required because of airway compromise a smaller bronchoscope is required.

Percutaneous Dilatation Tracheostomy

The need for long term mechanical ventilatory support is the most common indication for tracheostomy tube placement. Controversy exists on the benefits of early, less than, or equal to ten days or late greater than ten days for tracheostomy tube placement and discussion of

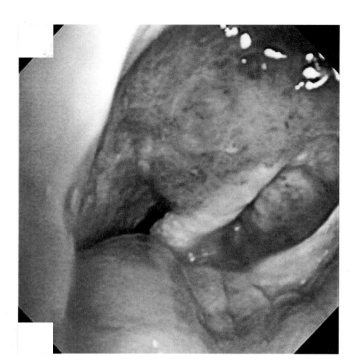

Figure 12.8 Subglotic intubation airway injury.

timing and patient selection is beyond the scope of this chapter. Percutaneous dilatation tracheostomy is increasingly being performed in the ICU at the bedside by intensivists, interventional pulmonologists, and surgeons the cost benefit and safety of this procedure in the ICU has been clearly established. The standard of care is for percutaneous dilatation tracheostomy to be guided by bronchoscopy to insure midline placement, and safety. The bronchoscopist stands at the head of the bed and inspects the airways and therapeutically aspirates secretions to insure good visualization and adequate oxygenation during the procedure, before the tracheostomy procedure is initiated the bronchoscopist is responsible for withdrawing the endo tracheal tube into the subglottic space this insures visualization of the needle insertion and minimizes the risk of endotracheal tube cuff rupture, by the needle, which could impact oxygenation and ventilation during the procedure. Once the bronchoscopist has positioned the endotracheal tube under direct visualization the procedure begins. Bronchoscopy allows for visualization of the needle insertion into the airway and insure midline insertion and that the cartilaginous rings are not injured. Subsequent dilation of the airway is visualized to insure there has been no injury to the posterior membrane. Once the tracheostomy tube has been placed the bronchoscopists inspect the airway through the newly inserted tracheostomy tube to insure there is no obstruction or bleeding.

Bronchoscopy can also serve as a tool to rapidly identify tracheostomy tubes that have become malpositioned. In patients with large-diameter necks or angioedema tracheostomy tubes can become partially displaced or fully displaced into the mediastinum. Large air leaks identified on the ventilator or new subcutaneous emphysema warrant airway inspection for tube position.

Bronchoscopy Emerging Technology in the ICU

Traditional bronchoscopy involves a significant capital investment in reusable bronchoscopes which require continuous cleaning and maintenance. There currently is an active interest in the development of disposable, single use, bronchoscopes. The theoretical advantage of disposable bronchoscopes is the elimination of scope damage or maintenance cost, no cleaning turnaround time, and elimination of infection control concerns. Current studies have looked at the use of disposable bronchoscopes in awake intubation in difficult airways and patients where there was concern with neck extension. Trials showed feasibility but failed to show superiority. As this technology evolves a potential role in critical care bronchoscopy may emerge.

Summary

Bronchoscopy is a tool that is now widely available in hospitals. The combined ability of direct visualization and sample acquisition makes it extremely useful in the diagnosis of chest diseases. Incorporating this potent tool in the critical care setting is becoming more and more regular. Bronchoscopy is a safe tool when appropriately applied in critically ill patients. Bronchoscopy extends our diagnostic capabilities in critically ill patients. In certain circumstances bronchoscopy improves safety in fragile critically ill patients.

The use of bronchoscopy in the intensive care unit requires good clinical judgment backed by appropriate training and a skilled supporting team.

Further Readings

Belanger A, Akulian J. Interventional pulmonology in the intensive care unit: percutaneous tracheostomy and gastrostomy. *Semin Respir Crit Care Med* 2014 Dec;35(6):744–750.

Cordonier C, Escudier E, Verra F, Brochard L, Bernaudin JF, Fleury-Feith J. Bronchoalveolar lavage during neutrapenic episodes: diagnostic yield and cellular pattern. *Eur Respir J* 1994;7:114–120.

Gruson D, Hilbert G, Valentino R, Vargas F, Chene G, Bebear C, Allery A, Pigneux A, Gbikpi-Benissan G, Cardinaud JP. Utility of fiberoptic bronchoscopy in neutropenic patients admitted to the intensive care unit with pulmonary infiltrates. *Crit Care Med* 2000;28:2224–2230.

Jackson SR, Ernst NE, Mueller EW, Butler KL. Utility of bronchoalveolar lavage for the diagnosis of ventilator-associated pneumonia in critically ill surgical patients. *Am J Surg* 2008;195:159–163.

Kelly SM, Marsh BR. Airway foreign bodies. *Chest Surg Clin N Am* 1996;6(2):253–276.

Kreider ME, Lipson D. Bronchoscopy for atelectasis in the ICU: a case report and review of the literature. *Chest* 2003;124:344–350.

Krugel V, Bathory I, Frascarolo P, Schoettker P. Comparison of the single-use ambu ascope 2 vs the conventional fiberscope for tracheal intubation in patients with cervical spine immobilization by a semirigid collar. *Anaesthesia* 2013;68:21–26.

Limper AH, Prakash UB. Trachealbroncheal foreign bodies in adults. *Ann Intern Med* 1990;112(8):604–609.

Marini JJ, Pierson DJ, Hudson LD. Acute lobar atelectasis: a prospective comparison of fiberoptic bronchoscopy and respiratory therapy. *Am Rev Respir Dis* 1979;119:971–978.

Papazian L, Colt HG, Scemama F, Martin C, Gouin F. Effects of consecutive protected specimen brushing and bronchoalveolar lavage on gas exchange and hemodynamics in ventilated patients. *Chest* 1993;104:1548–1552.

Peikert T, Rana S, Edell ES. Safety, diagnostic yield and therapeutic implications of flexible bronchoscopy in patients with febrile neutrapenia and pulmonary infiltrates. *Mayo Clin Proc* 2005;80(11):1414–1420.

Rafanan AL, Mehta AC. Adult airway foreign body removal. *Whats New? Clin Chest Med* 2001;22(2):319–330.

Steinberg KP, Mitchell DR, Maunder RJ, Milberg JA, Whitcomb ME. Safety of bronchoalveolar lavage in patients with adult respiratory distress syndrome. *Am Rev Respir Dis* 1993;148:556–561.

Weiss S, Hert R, Gianola FJ, Clark JG, Crawford SW. Complications of fiberoptic bronchoscopy in thrombocytopenic patients. *Chest* 1993;104:1025–1028.

White P, Bonacum JT, Miller CB. Utility of fiberoptic bronchoscopy in bone marrow transplant patients. *Bone Marrow Transplant* 1997;20:681–687.

Zollner F. Gustav killian father of bronchoscopy. *Arch Otolaryngol* 1965;82:656–659.

Chapter 13

Basic Endobronchial Ultrasound

Maren Schuhmann

Introduction

Mediastinal lymph node enlargement can occur in several benign diseases such as sarcoidosis and tuberculosis and also in malignant diseases such as lung cancer, lymphoma, or metastases of other primary origin. Lymph node staging is important with regards to the therapeutic and prognostic implications this carries for the patient.

Computer tomography is often the first staging tool when lung cancer is suspected and lymph nodes at a size of over 1 cm are deemed suspicious for metastases. The sensitivity and specificity of using CT alone is low especially in lymph nodes under 2 cm. The prognostic accuracy increases with the use of PET-CT but even then it is important to sample enlarged lymph nodes and obtain a tissue diagnosis before proceeding to potentially curative surgery. For many years mediastinoscopy has been the gold standard for the investigation and staging of the mediastinum. But it is an invasive and expensive procedure with associated morbidity and mortality. Over the last few years endosonography has been increasingly used in the staging of lung cancer as well as the diagnosis of unexplained mediastinal lymphadenopathy.

Gastroenterologists have been using endosonography for many years in the staging of oesphageal carcinoma and in the 1990s the same technique was adapted as a diagnostic tool in the airways. EBUS and EUS (endoesophageal ultrasound) are these days routinely used and allow for the visualization and sampling of mediastinal lymph nodes that lie adjacent to the trachea or oesophagus respectively. They are not only used in the diagnosis of benign diseases such as sarcoidosis, tuberculosis, or inflammatory processes but also in malignant diseases. With EUS the left adrenal gland and lesions in the left lobe of the liver can also be sampled to allow for metastatic staging.

EBUS Scope

An EBUS (endobronchial ultrasound) scope is similar to a regular scope and uses video and fiberoptic technologies to obtain a picture. In addition to a regular bronchoscope a curved linear array 7.5–12 MHz ultrasonic transducer is mounted at its distal end (Figure 13.1). Models are available through different companies and currently the smallest available diameter is 6.3 mm with a 2.2-mm working channel.

The endoscopic picture is supplied by a 30° angle optic and hence introducing this bronchoscope past the vocal cords can be a little more challenging than a normal video-bronchoscope at the beginning. The EBUS scope is wider than a regular bronchoscope and access to the more distal airways can be difficult. The distal ultrasonic tip can be fitted with a water inflatable balloon to improve contact with the mucosal wall and visualization of

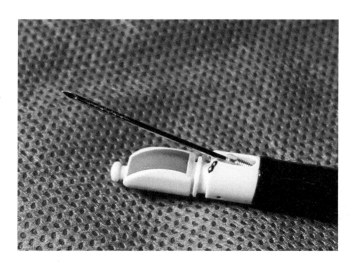

Figure 13.1 Distal tip of a EBUS bronchoscope.

the structures lying beyond. This can be useful when mucosal contact is otherwise poor or cartilage is overlying the targeted lymph node. Use of the balloon can be particularly useful in the trachea when the procedure is performed under light sedation only to avoid coughing.

By pushing the distal tip against the mucosal wall the ultrasonic picture can be obtained. The ultrasound image is obtained with a dedicated ultrasound processor and color Doppler mode can also be displayed in order to differentiate vascular structure from solid tissue (Figure 13.2).

Identified structures can be visually enlarged and measured for documentation during the procedure. The EBUS scope allows for the visualization of lymph nodes but also for tumour infiltration or imaging of other structures adjacent to the trachea or main bronchi.

When a lymph node is identified it should be measured and its echogeneity should be documented. Lymph nodes of under 1 cm, of oval shape with visible presence of the hilar structure are more likely to be benign whereas lymph nodes over 1 cm with low echogeneity and necrosis tend to be malignant nodes. It is important to remember however that echo features are not absolute measures and can only provide guidance with regards to which node to biopsy.

Once a structure has been identified it can be punctured with a dedicated 21 or 22 gauge needle under continued direct visualization. The needle is passed into the working channel and secured in place. It is important to adjust the sheath containing the needle for it to be just visible in the endoscopic picture. This has to be performed with the distal tip in a straightened position in order to avoid damage to the distal bronchoscope. Once the needle is advanced into the working channel the distal tip becomes stiffer and may be more difficult to flex. The lymph node is punctured under direct visualization and can be seen on the endoscopic as well as the ultrasound picture (Figure 13.3). A stylet within the needle avoids sampling of bronchial mucosa during the puncture and has to be removed after puncturing the lymph node.

Suction is applied via a 20 ml vacutainer syringe. Aspirations can also be performed by simply withdrawing the stylet a few centimeters and aspirating with the use of capillary forces

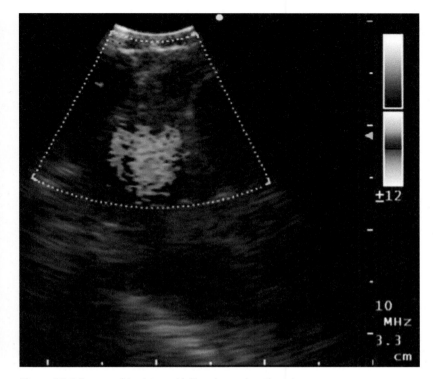

Figure 13.2 Sonographic picture with Doppler mode activated.

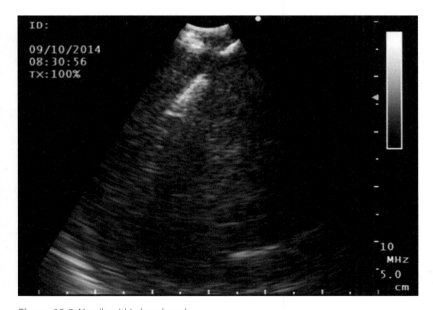

Figure 13.3 Needle within lymph node.

within the needle. The use of the vacutainer syringe in comparison to not using suction has been studied by Casal et al and no difference in sample yield or quality has been found.

During the aspiration it is recommended to advance and withdraw the needle within the lymph node several times in order to obtain an adequate sample. No data has been published as to the recommended amount of times the lymph node should be traversed, but experts recommend approximately 8–20 times. Once this has been performed, the suction is removed, the needle withdrawn back into the sheath and secured, and the sheath and needle are removed from the working channel. The samples are then transferred onto glass slides or into formalin for a cell block.

It is recommended to puncture lymph nodes at least three times to obtain enough material for smears and a cell block. Routinely, two punctures are performed for cytosmear and one is expelled into formalin for a cytospin and cell block. If adequate samples are obtained these are often sufficient to perform analyses including immunohistochemical stains. If samples are small or dry aspiration is performed it is recommended to sample the node several more times. Close cooperation with the local cytopathologist is recommended in order to supply good samples and achieve the best results.

Some centers may have access to rapid on site evaluation (ROSE) or physicians may perform this themselves. ROSE has been shown to decrease the number of punctures required if core samples were obtained hence decreasing the intervention time. Lee et al were able to show that 75 percent of EBUS TBNA contained core tissue allowing for molecular testing including EGFR and ALK mutation analysis.

EBUS bronchoscopy can be performed under local anesthesia, mild sedation, or general anesthesia. Coughing can make it difficult for beginners to obtain adequate pictures and more sedation may be required. Yarmus et al compared moderate versus deep sedation and found that the diagnostic yield as well as number of lymph nodes sampled was greater in procedures performed under deep rather than only moderate sedation. Moderate sedation for this procedure is generally well tolerated by patients.

Anatomy

When using an EBUS scope it is important to understand the mediastinal anatomy and the areas which can be accessed by the EBUS scope. It is important to apply a systematic approach to the different lymph node stations in order to avoid oversight. Especially in patients with (suspected) lung cancer adequate lymph node staging is important to choose the most appropriate form of therapy for the patient.

The modified Mountain–Dresler lymph node map presents a good starting point to identify the different lymph node stations (Figure 13.4).

EBUS can reach the high mediastinal nodes (station 1), the upper paratracheal nodes (station 2), lower paratracheal nodes (station 4), subcarinal nodes (station 7) as well as hilar nodes (stations 10 and 11). In some patients stations 12 and/or 13 can also be reached. Endo-oesophageal ultrasound can reach positions 2, 4, 7, 8, and 9 as well as the left adrenal gland and the left lobe of the liver.

When performing a lymph node staging in suspected or known cancer patients it is important to initially sample the N3 lymph nodes, followed by N2, and then N1 in order to avoid contamination.

Whilst performing EBUS TBNA it is easiest to use anatomical landmarks visible in the endoscopic picture as well as vascular markings identified by endobronchial ultrasound.

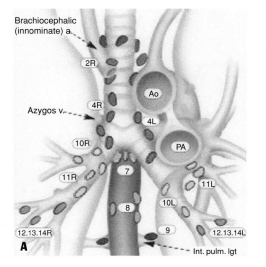
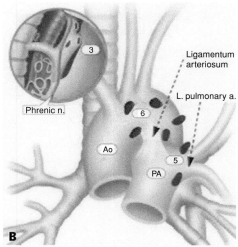

Figure 13.4 Mountain–Dresler lymph node map.

Station 12R: The EBUS scope is advanced into the lower lobe bronchus proximal to branching of the lower basal bronchus. Station 12R is adjacent to the interlobular pulmonary artery.

Station 11R: Withdraw EBUS scope into the intermediate bronchus, turn clockwise, and press the tip to the upper lobe carina. Station 11R can be seen adjacent to the interlobar pulmonary artery.

Station 10R: Move the tip of the EBUS scope into the right upper lobe bronchus, turn clockwise to a 3 o'clock position, and withdraw the bronchoscope slightly.

Lymph node stations 10R and 4R are separated by the azygos vein. The lower border of the azygos vein indicates the top of lymph node station 10R, anything above the lower border is declared as lymph node station 4R

Station 4R: Withdraw the EBUS scope from here further and rotate slightly anti-clockwise. The station can be found just above the level of the main carina.

Station 2R: On withdrawing the bronchoscope further in the trachea keeping it in a 2–3 o'clock position, station 2R can be visualized.

Lymph node station 1R is difficult to visualize.

Station 12L: As on the contralateral side the bronchoscope is advanced into the basal segment and rotated clockwise and anticlockwise slightly. These nodes can be difficult to identify.

Station 11L: On withdrawing the bronchoscope and pushing it against the carina between the upper and lower lobe the lymph node can be visualized next to the pulmonary artery.

Station 10L: Retracting the bronchoscope into the left main bronchus into a 10 o'clock position lymph node 10L is seen in close proximity to the pulmonary artery.

Station 4L: The bronchoscope is withdrawn further in the left main bronchus and turned anticlockwise to a 10 o'clock position at the level of the main carina. Lymph node station 4L lies between the aorta and the left main pulmonary artery.

Station 2L: In the upper trachea turn the bronchoscope anticlockwise into a 11 o'clock position. Lymph node station 2L lies above the aortic arch (Figure 13.5).

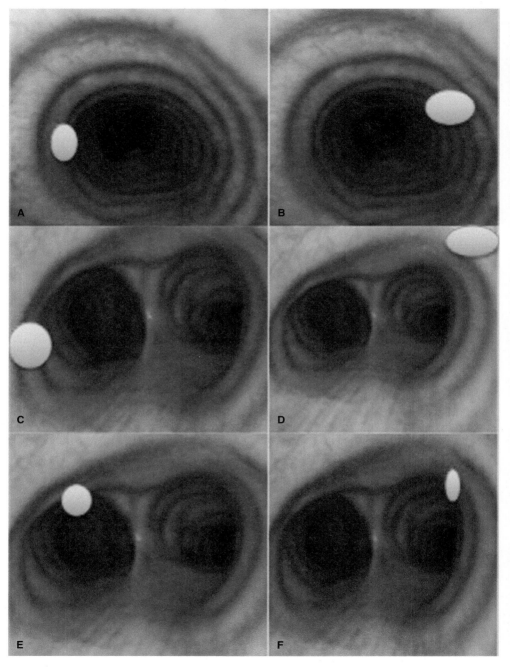

Figure 13.5 a–ef Endobronchial equivalent of lymph node stations 2L **(A)**, 2R **(B)**, 4L **(C)**, 4R **(D)**, 10L **(E)**, and 10R **(F)**

Complications

EBUS TBNA is a very safe procedure and complications observed are very rare. In a meta-analysis by Gu et al an overall complication rate of 0.15 percent was recorded and rare complications such as mediastinitis, lung abscess, pericarditis, and pneumothorax have been reported as case series only. Infectious complications were found when puncturing cystic lesions and antibiotics are recommended should a puncture be performed via EUS. EBUS TBNA was also found to be safe to perform in patients taking clopidogrel although this was a small case series only. As with regular bronchoscopy other complications such as infection, transient fever, haemoptysis, and others can also occur.

Damage to the bronchoscope by erroneous use of the needle or other handling mistakes can be a very expensive complication and regular training by the bronchoscope provider for the whole team involved with handling this device is recommended.

Learning Curve

EBUS TBNA takes time to learn under experienced guidance in order to fully understand the ultrasonographic pictures not seen in regular bronchoscopy. There exists no consensus in the national and international guidelines as to how best to train physicians in this technique. Learning curves have been studied and one Australian study reported that the diagnostic yield improved significantly by 20 procedures but 50 procedures were required to reach the peak of diagnostic yield. Another trial recommended performing 13 procedures under supervision to be able to perform the procedure safely and obtain an adequate yield. Different learning models have been proposed and Konge et al published data on the use of virtual reality bronchoscopy simulators to assess the performance in order to set a standard training prior to "real-life" bronchoscopy. Skills learned on simulators appear to be transferrable to a clinical setting. Larger trials are necessary here but more training opportunities need to be implemented since the technique is becoming more ubiquitous.

Literature Review

First published use and results for EBUS TBNA was in 2003 by Mark Krasnik and 2004 by Yasufuku. Since then the technique and its use has spread and multiple studies have been published and meta-analyses summarized the results. Gu et al published a meta-analysis with 1299 patients with lung cancer showing a pooled sensitivity of 0.93 and a pooled specificity of 1.00. A sensitivity of 0.94 was shown for patients who had an EBUS-TBNA based on CT or positron emission tomography (PET)-CT positive results. The sensitivity and accuracy of EBUS-TBNA for the prediction of lymph node involvement was superior to using CT or PET. Even when comparing EBUS TBNA staging to staging with mediastinoscopy its sensitivity and accuracy is very similar prompting national and international guidelines to change their diagnostic pathway to make use of EBUS TBNA prior to subjecting a patient to the more invasive procedure of a mediastinoscopy. EBUS TBNA has fewer complications than mediastinoscopy and can be performed as a day case procedure.

A complete mediastinal staging however cannot be accomplished by the use of EBUS alone since not all lymph nodes are accessible via the bronchial tree. EBUS needs to be combined with EUS in order to cover most mediastinal lymph node stations as well as the left adrenal gland. Stations 5 and 6 however are only accessed by anterior mediastinoscopy.

Annema et al were able to show that combined endosonography with surgical staging had a greater sensitivity for mediastinal lymph node metastases than surgical staging alone.

The EBUS scope can be used endobronchially as well as via the esophagus and this "one scope approach" has been shown to be feasible and to provide a better diagnostic accuracy than either procedure alone. Depending on the size of the patient the left adrenal gland can be reached with the regular EBUS scope as well.

When comparing the 21 and 22 gauge needle to perform EBUS TBNA no difference was found in a retrospective study with regards to the diagnostic yield. A transbronchial needle forceps has also been evaluated and found a higher diagnostic yield compared to a 21G needle. These may be useful in diagnosing benign diseases or in the diagnosis of lymphoma but more data is needed here. 19G needles as well as "tru-cut" needles are being produced by different manufacturers to aid diagnosis in benign disease and lymphoma. No trials have been published as yet comparing these to the standard available 21 and 22G needles.

In the diagnosis of benign mediastinal lymphadenopathy due to suspected sarcoidosis a prospective randomized trial compared the use of EBUS TBNA with transbronchial biopsies. It found a diagnostic yield for the detection of granulomas of 80 percent with EBUS TBNA and only 53 percent with transbronchial biopsies and this technique should be employed before resorting to mediastinoscopy. The use of EBUS in suspected tuberculosis is less well established but one multi-center case series describing 156 patients with a diagnosis of TB associated lymphadenopathy reports a sensitivity and accuracy of 94 percent.

In the diagnosis of lymphoma larger specimens are often required to diagnose the exact subtype and grading. A study by Steinfort et al evaluated EBUS TBNA in lymphoma and found a diagnostic sensitivity of 76 percent but some of these patients required further biopsy reducing the sensitivity to 57 percent. EBUS TBNA should not be considered the first diagnostic approach in suspected lymphoma but can identify a proportion of patients with the disease.

Of course EBUS TBNA samples are smaller than samples obtained by mediastinoscopy, potentially resulting in more false negative samples. Hence current guidelines recommend mediastinoscopy following a negative EBUS TBNA result should there still be concern about the lymph node stations. Performing EBUS TBNA prior to mediastinoscopy reduces the need for more invasive procedures and unnecessary thoracotomies.

Summary

EBUS provides a real time assessment and sampling of enlarged mediastinal lymph nodes and is a safe tool in the diagnosis of benign and malignant diseases. It is becoming increasingly important in the diagnosis and staging of lung cancer as well as the diagnosis of benign diseases. Published trials confirm EBUS TBNA as the first line investigation of choice accepting that there may still be a need for more invasive testing if the results are negative. More randomized trials are required particularly in the field of benign disease and lymphoma.

Further Readings

Annema JT, van Meerbeeck JP, Rintoul RC, Dooms C, Deschepper E, Dekkers OM, et al. Mediastinoscopy vs endosonography for mediastinal nodal staging of lung cancer: a randomized trial. *JAMA*. 2010 Nov 24;304(20):2245–2252.

Casal RF, Staerkel GA, Ost D, Almeida FA, Uzbeck MH, Eapen GA, et al. Randomized clinical trial of endobronchial ultrasound needle biopsy with and without aspiration. *Chest*. 2012 Sep;142(3): 568–573.

Ernst A, Anantham D, Eberhardt R, Krasnik M, Herth FJ. Diagnosis of mediastinal adenopathy-real-time endobronchial ultrasound guided needle aspiration versus mediastinoscopy. *J Thorac Oncol*. 2008 Jun;3(6):577–582.

Fujiwara T, Yasufuku K, Nakajima T, Chiyo M, Yoshida S, Suzuki M, et al. The utility of sonographic features during endobronchial ultrasound-guided transbronchial needle aspiration for lymph node staging in patients with lung cancer: a standard endobronchial ultrasound image classification system. *Chest*. 2010 Sep;138(3):641–647.

Gu P, Zhao YZ, Jiang LY, Zhang W, Xin Y, Han BH. Endobronchial ultrasound-guided transbronchial needle aspiration for staging of lung cancer: a systematic review and meta-analysis. *Eur J Cancer*. 2009 May;45(8):1389–1396.

Herth FJ, Schuler H, Gompelmann D, Kahn N, Gasparini S, Ernst A, et al. Endobronchial ultrasound-guided lymph node biopsy with transbronchial needle forceps: a pilot study. *Eur Respir J*. 2012 Feb;39(2):373–377.

Hwangbo B, Lee GK, Lee HS, Lim KY, Lee SH, Kim HY, et al. Transbronchial and transesophageal fine-needle aspiration using an ultrasound bronchoscope in mediastinal staging of potentially operable lung cancer. *Chest*. 2010 Oct;138(4):795–802.

Konge L, Annema J, Clementsen P, Minddal V, Vilmann P, Ringsted C. Using virtual-reality simulation to assess performance in endobronchial ultrasound. *Respiration*. 2013 Jan;86(1): 59–65.

Krasnik M, Vilmann P, Larsen SS, Jacobsen GK. Preliminary experience with a new method of endoscopic transbronchial real time ultrasound guided biopsy for diagnosis of mediastinal and hilar lesions. *Thorax*. 2003 Dec;58(12):1083–1086.

Lee HS, Lee GK, Kim MS, Lee JM, Kim HY, Nam BH, et al. Real-time endobronchial ultrasound-guided transbronchial needle aspiration in mediastinal staging of non-small cell lung cancer: how many aspirations per target lymph node station? *Chest*. 2008 Aug;134(2): 368–374.

Navani N, Molyneaux PL, Breen RA, Connell DW, Jepson A, Nankivell M, et al. Utility of endobronchial ultrasound-guided transbronchial needle aspiration in patients with tuberculous intrathoracic lymphadenopathy: a multicentre study. *Thorax*. 2011 Oct;66(10):889–893.

Polkowski M, Larghi A, Weynand B, Boustiere C, Giovannini M, Pujol B, et al. Learning, techniques, and complications of endoscopic ultrasound (EUS)-guided sampling in gastroenterology: European Society of Gastrointestinal Endoscopy (ESGE) Technical Guideline. *Endoscopy*. 2012 Feb;44(2):190–206.

Stather DR, MacEachern P, Chee A, Tremblay A. Safety of endobronchial ultrasound-guided transbronchial needle aspiration for patients taking clopidogrel: a report of 12 consecutive cases. *Respiration*. 2012 Apr;83(4):330–334.

Stather DR, MacEachern P, Chee A, Dumoulin E, Tremblay A. Evaluation of clinical endobronchial ultrasound skills following clinical versus simulation training. *Respirology*. 2012 Feb;17(2): 291–299.

Steinfort DP, Irving LB. Patient satisfaction during endobronchial ultrasound-guided transbronchial needle aspiration performed under conscious sedation. *Respir Care*. 2010 Jun;55(6): 702–706.

Steinfort DP, Hew MJ, Irving LB. Bronchoscopic evaluation of the mediastinum using endobronchial ultrasound: a description of the first 216 cases carried out at an Australian tertiary hospital. *Intern Med J*. 2011 Dec;41(12):815–824.

Steinfort DP, Conron M, Tsui A, Pasricha SR, Renwick WE, Antippa P, et al. Endobronchial ultrasound-guided transbronchial needle aspiration for the evaluation of suspected lymphoma. *J Thorac Oncol*. 2010 Jun;5(6):804–809.

Toloza EM, Harpole L, McCrory DC. Noninvasive staging of non-small cell lung cancer: a review of the current evidence. *Chest*. 2003 Jan;123(1 Suppl):137S–146S.

von Bartheld MB, Dekkers OM, Szlubowski A, Eberhardt R, Herth FJ, in 't Veen JC, et al. Endosonography vs conventional bronchoscopy for the diagnosis of sarcoidosis: the GRANULOMA randomized clinical trial. *JAMA*. 2013 Jun 19;309(23):2457–2464.

Wahidi MM, Hulett C, Pastis N, Shepherd RW, Shofer SL, Mahmood K, et al. Learning experience of linear endobronchial ultrasound among pulmonary trainees. *Chest*. 2014 Mar 1;145(3):574–578.

Yarmus LB, Akulian JA, Gilbert C, Mathai SC, Sathiyamoorthy S, Sahetya S, et al. Comparison of moderate versus deep sedation for endobronchial ultrasound transbronchial needle aspiration. *Ann Am Thorac Soc*. 2013 Apr;10(2):121–126.

Yarmus LB, Akulian J, Lechtzin N, Yasin F, Kamdar B, Ernst A, et al. Comparison of 21-gauge and 22-gauge aspiration needle in endobronchial ultrasound-guided transbronchial needle aspiration: results of the American College of Chest Physicians Quality Improvement Registry, Education, and Evaluation Registry. *Chest*. 2013 Apr;143(4):1036–1043.

Yasufuku K, Chhajed PN, Sekine Y, Nakajima T, Chiyo M, Iyoda A, et al. Endobronchial ultrasound using a new convex probe: a preliminary study on surgically resected specimens. *Oncol Rep*. 2004 Feb;11(2):293–296.

Yasufuku K, Nakajima T, Motoori K, Sekine Y, Shibuya K, Hiroshima K, et al. Comparison of endobronchial ultrasound, positron emission tomography, and CT for lymph node staging of lung cancer. *Chest*. 2006 Sep;130(3):710–718.

Bronchoscopy in the Lung Transplant Patient

Anne Fuhlbrigge

Lung transplantation has rapidly evolved since the first operation in the early 1960s and has become an established treatment for a variety of patients with end-stage lung disease. Bronchoscopy is an essential tool in the diagnosis and management of lung transplant recipients. In the following chapter we will outline four areas in which bronchoscopy plays a critical role in the care of patients undergoing lung transplantation; evaluation of potential lung donors, surveillance for acute rejection, evaluation and treatment among lung transplant recipients presenting with new symptoms or deteriorating respiratory function, Visualization of the anastomosis and management of airway complications.

The Role of Bronchoscopy in the Assessment of Potential Lung Donors

Flexible bronchoscopy is an essential part of the evaluation of all potential lung donors.

Bronchoscopy can assess for evidence of lung injury, inflammation, aspiration, and infection. If bronchoscopy is normal, without anatomic abnormality, endobronchial lesions or secretions, acceptance of the organ for donation is appropriate. Only 33 percent of persons meeting criteria for brain death and being considered for donation will have a normal bronchoscopy. A normal bronchoscopy is not a requirement for accepting a potential lung donor; yet, the findings on flexible bronchoscopy can help differentiate donors acceptable for donation from donors that should be rejected.

Detailed Inspection of the Anatomy

An important finding during bronchoscopy is the presence of anatomic variations that influence the operative procedure and potential use of the organ. As an example, the author has encountered a potential donor in which the orifice for the RUL was located very proximally in relation to the carina making anastomosis difficult without sacrificing the RUL during the procedure. Decisions regarding specific anatomic variants and how they might impact the use of potential donor organs should be routinely discussed with the accepting transplant surgeon.

Obtaining Microbiologic Samples

Aspiration and pneumonia are common in potential donors, yet the presence of mucopurulent secretions among potential donors without clear clinical evidence of pneumonia and with a clear CXR is fairly common. Bronchoscopy can guide in the selection of organs in such cases. If extensive endobronchial inflammation is seen or if extensive secretions emanate

Post-Transplant Bronchoscopy Schedule

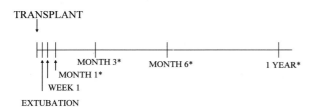

Figure 14.1 Sample schedule for routine surveillance bronchoscopy at a single lung transplant center. Surveillance bronchoscopy to assess anastomotic healing and to aid in pulmonary clearance is performed prior to extubation and at 1 week post-transplant. Routine surveillance bronchoscopy with transbronchial biopsy is performed at 1, 3, 6, and 12 months post-transplant.

*Transbronchial biopsy

from the distal segments that do not readily clear, the donor may have suffered a significant aspiration event and despite a clear CXR may be developing an infection that precludes accepting the lung for donation. Alternatively, if the endobronchial mucosa is normal in appearance and the secretions are easily suctioned clear during the examination, the potential donor lungs are likely appropriate for use. In this situation, bronchoscopy can also be used to obtain specimens to facilitate targeted antimicrobial therapy in the recipient during the immediate postoperative period. There is debate regarding the importance of a positive gram stain in the selection of donors for transplantation but prior studies have shown no correlation between a positive donor gram stain and subsequent postoperative pneumonia in the recipient.

Surveillance Bronchoscopy

Close surveillance of the allograft is the key to a successful transplant outcome. In many centers routine surveillance bronchoscopy at predetermined time intervals for the evaluation of acute rejection is a central component of this surveillance (Figure 14.1).

Recent surveys of transplant programs across the United States and internationally, documented that over 50 percent of programs perform surveillance procedures. Transbronchial biopsy (TBBx) is the gold standard for the diagnosis of acute rejection with sensitivities in the range of 93 percent reported for acute rejection, however studies have shown a false negative rate of between 15 and 28 percent. Variation in yield may be related to technique as published reports have varied in their sampling methods from three pieces in one lobe to 17 pieces from both lungs. At most US centers only one lung is biopsied to avoid the risk of bilateral pneumothoraces (PTX). The decision regarding the number of biopsies is a balance between obtaining enough biopsies to achieve an adequate diagnostic yield without an unnecessarily high risk of complications. The consensus recommendation is that a specimen containing five pieces of alveolated lung parenchyma, each with a minimum of 100 alveoli and bronchioles is acceptable to minimize the risk of sampling error and false negative results and optimize yield.

Lung transplant recipients are at highest risk of acute rejection in the first 6–12 months following lung transplant. On the other hand, chronic rejection is rarely seen before six months. In addition, the presence of chronic rejection in biopsies does not correlate well with functional status and the diagnostic yield from flexible bronchoscopy in chronic rejection is much lower than with acute rejection. Therefore many lung transplant centers do not perform surveillance bronchoscopy with TBBx after the first year. The diagnosis and staging of chronic lung allograft dysfunction, bronchiolitis obliterans syndrome (BOS), are based on clinical criteria (FEV_1) and are defined as graft deterioration due to progressive airway disease for which there is no evidence of another superimposed process. Bronchoscopy does play an important role in excluding other treatable causes of graft dysfunction but cannot routinely confirm the diagnosis of chronic rejection.

The use of routine surveillance TBBx remains an area of debate among clinicians. Proponents underscore the frequency of unexpected findings during surveillance bronchoscopy seen in up to one quarter to one third of specimens during the first 400 days, which influence management. This is confirmed by a program that performed surveillance bronchoscopy among clinically healthy lung transplant recipients and found significant abnormalities in a large proportion of patients; 39 percent had some degree of acute rejection, 14 percent had evidence of CMV, 18 percent had nonspecific findings with only 24 percent being read as normal. Importantly, it has been demonstrated that asymptomatic mild acute rejection, when left untreated, can progress to symptomatic higher grade rejection, and that patients who experience multiple low grade rejection episodes in the first year of transplant may develop earlier onset chronic rejection, independent of whether they go on to develop higher grades of rejection, suggesting these patients may warrant more aggressive immunosuppression. Finally, the importance of follow-up bronchoscopy after a documented episode of rejection is highlighted, where persistent rejection was found in many cases that required further treatment.

In contrast, opponents of routine surveillance highlight the lack of data showing a significant difference in long term outcome, including mortality, among patients in whom surveillance bronchoscopy is performed, compared to patients in whom bronchoscopy is only performed when clinically indicated by symptoms or fall in lung function. In addition, opponents highlight the costs of repeated procedures and the associated risk of complications. No randomized controlled trials have examined this issue and the available data to guide this decision comes from retrospective, nonrandomized studies with their inherent limitations.

Diagnostic Bronchoscopy for Evaluation of Clinical Deterioration

Diagnostic bronchoscopy can provide valuable information in lung transplant recipients that present with new respiratory symptoms or a decline in functional status. Pulmonary infections in lung transplant patients can be difficult to diagnose. The presenting signs and symptoms are very similar between infectious and noninfectious complications of transplantation. DeVito Dabbs and colleagues found no significant differences in the severity or type of symptoms between patients that were diagnosed with infection vs. those found to have rejection. Bronchoscopy with BAL, and TBBx play a critical role in differentiating these two entities when interpretation of the biopsy is made in light of the entire clinical, microbiologic, and radiographic picture. Some reports highlight the role of cell counts and differentials counts in the management of lung transplant recipients but the routine use of this has not been adopted in all centers.

Infection represents a leading cause of death in the first year after transplant, with the rate of infection being higher among lung transplant patients compared with other solid organ transplants. The reasons for this increased risk of infection are several, but a primary reason is the required suppression of humoral and cell medicated immunity by immunosuppressant therapy. The dosing of immunosuppressant medications is highest during the first year secondary to a higher risk of rejection during this same period. Therefore, the balance of competing risks, infection and rejection, is more difficult in the first year (Figure 14.2).

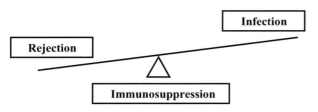

Figure 14.2 Illustration of the pivotal role immunosuppressive therapy plays in the balance between the risk of rejection and risk of infection among lung transplant recipients. This balance is particularly difficult in the first year post-transplant.

Other changes in the innate defense of lung transplant patients play a role in the increased risk of infection. In the immediate postoperative period, lung transplant recipients have a blunted cough reflex due to postoperative pain and the denervation of the lung that occurs. This contributes to poor clearance of respiratory secretions and the potential for microaspiration, which is aggravated in many patients by postoperative gastroparesis. In addition, poor lymphatic drainage, impaired mucociliary clearance secondary to ischemic injury to the mucosa, and narrowing of the anastomosis with sloughing of devitalized cartilage can all impair pulmonary hygiene and secretion clearance, leading to the high incidence of bacterial infections after lung transplantation.

Secondary to inadequate secretion clearance, bronchoscopy is a valuable therapeutic tool in the postoperative period, discussed further (Therapeutic bronchoscopy). Of note the blunted cough reflex among lung transplant patients can have an advantage, reducing the amount of topical anesthesia needed within the airway. However, it is important to note that among patients with a single lung transplant, the cough reflex is intact in the native lung.

Bacterial infections occur most frequently, with 43–63 percent of infections following lung transplant secondary to bacterial pathogens. However viral (23–31 percent), fungal (10–14 percent), and other (4–10 percent) opportunistic pathogens including mycobacterial disease, *Nocardia, Actinomyces, Legionella*, and *Listeria moncytogenes* must be considered. Although, routine gram stain, and culture are essential components in the evaluation of a change in clinical status, other specimens should be tailored to risk factors and/or exposures known in a given patient. *Aspergillus* is commonly isolated during bronchoscopy among lung transplant patients but may be transient and associated with necrotic tissue found at the anastomotic site without true invasion. *Pneumocystis carinii* is a potential opportunist infection following lung transplantation but has been virtually eliminated by the routine use of prophylaxis. In the era before prophylaxis, infection was reported in up to 88 percent of heart and lung transplant recipients.

Even if bronchoscopy is performed, a pathogen is not always identified in the setting of clinical infection, secondary to initiating antibiotic treatment prior to the procedure. In addition, the sensitivity of bronchoscopy for diagnosing rejection is dependent on technique. In a study of bronchoscopy among patients with new respiratory symptoms utilizing TBBx, BAL, and protected specimen brush (PSB), only 17.5 percent of 114 diagnoses of bacterial infection were established using BAL. The diagnostic yield increased with the use of PSB.

Performing bronchoscopy in lung transplant patients is similar to that in non-transplant patients. Lung transplant recipients typically undergo multiple bronchoscopies during their post-transplant course and effective sedation is important to allow a safe and beneficial procedure and insure the patient is willing to undergo repeated procedures, it is important to note that patients with Cystic fibrosis, who make up a significant proportion of lung transplant patients, tend to require higher doses of sedative medication for the procedure. Propofol can be a useful alternative if adequate sedation cannot be achieved with usual doses of midazolam and fentanyl. A common observation among lung transplant patients is a suppressed cough reflex in the bronchial tree of their allograft, likely related to the denervation of the graft at the time of transplant, reducing the need for topical airway anesthesia. Similar to bronchoscopy performed in non-transplant patients, complications of TBBx in lung transplant recipients include pneumothorax (1–3 percent), pulmonary hemorrhage (10–15 percent), arrhythmia (2 percent), upper airway obstruction requiring intervention (10 percent), and cardiopulmonary arrest and death (0.01 percent). As with any procedure, the risk of not performing a diagnostic procedure and proceeding without additional information that may influence management must be weighed against the risk of the procedure.

The risk of bleeding has been reported to be higher in lung transplant recipients compared with that reported in other populations and appears to be independent of traditional bleeding risks, including coagulation parameters, platelet count, serum creatinine, or use of aspirin or immunosuppressive drugs. It is also not correlated with the presence of acute rejection, BOS, the number of biopsies taken or time since transplant. Improved bleeding rates among lung transplant patients has been shown after implementing a standardized protocol of (1) desmopressin for BUN >30, (2) avoidance of TBBx in patient with known pulmonary hypertension, and (3) withholding antiplatelet agents before the procedure. The contribution of each to the improved bleeding rates was not evaluated. Some programs, including ours, perform all procedures utilizing endotracheal intubation (without balloon deployed). This protocol can provide improved access to the airway during the procedure. In addition, it allows easy access to the airway for debridement when necessary in the early post-transplant period. Finally, lung transplant patients may be at a higher risk for desaturation during the procedure and performing the procedure following intubation can avoid upper airway obstruction, which is commonly implicated in desaturation events.

Visualization of the Anastomosis and Management of Airway Complications

Bronchoscopy is the gold standard in the diagnosis of airway complications and instrumental in their management. The most common anastomotic airway complications include; stenosis, bronchomalacia, granulation tissue, anastomotic dehiscence, bronchial fistulae (bronchomediastinal, bronchovascular, and bronchopleural), and anastomotic infections.

Airway complications are relatively common among lung transplant recipients and diagnosis of problems with the integrity of the anastomosis is critical in the management of lung transplant patients. Early studies suggested findings of airway complications in as many as 57 percent of patients. Changes in donor lung procurement, operative techniques, and postoperative management have lowered this risk, resulting in lower rates of airway complications reported in more recent reports (12–17 percent). The majority of airway complications involve the larger central airways and in particular the bronchial anastomosis. The bronchial artery circulation is lost during the harvest of the donor lung and limited bronchial artery revascularization from the recipient bronchial artery may take 3–4 weeks to occur after transplantation. During this time, the airway is dependent on retrograde low pressure flow from the poorly oxygenated blood available in the pulmonary artery and the risk of ischemia of the proximal donor bronchus (area just distal to the anastomosis in the recipient) is high. The majority of airways will suffer ischemic injury to the airway wall and display inflammation and erythema of some degree after transplantation. The severity of this process correlates with the risk of more serious airway complications. Several systems, such as the Courad, TEGLA, and MDS grading systems, have been proposed to standardize the reporting of airway complications. However, no universally accepted classification system has been adopted which contributes to the variable incidence rates of reported airway complications. In the immediate postoperative period bronchoscopy plays a role in monitoring the anastomosis and in helping with pulmonary hygiene and management of secretions. Early diagnosis of poor anastomotic healing can help in targeting a patient for close surveillance and determining the need for continued antimicrobial therapy secondary to airway infection. Changes in the innate defense in lung transplant patients discussed earlier, promote injury to the airway, which can lead to an increased risk of infection. In addition, poor lymphatic drainage in the transplanted lung dictates that patients are aggressively diuresed in the perioperative period; this can cause secretions to be thick and tenacious making mobilization difficult. Bronchoscopy, during this early period, can help clear blood clots, thick tenacious secretions, and necrotic tissue to help maintain a patent airway. In the majority of cases this can be completed with a flexible bronchoscope using forceps. Less commonly debridement in the OR using laser, cryotherapy, or a rigid bronchoscope may be necessary.

Airway Stenosis

Stenosis is a late complication felt to be secondary to healing of early anastomotic complications or the result of chronic rejection. Stenosis may cause secretion retention which may predispose to recurrent infections. Bronchoscopy can aid in the management of bronchial stenosis and may include mechanical dilation, bronchoscopic airway debridement, and ablative therapy using laser, cryotherapy, argon plasma coagulation (APC), brachytherapy, electrocautery, cryotherapy, and photodynamic therapy. Additional approaches that have been used in the treatment of benign airway stenosis include injection of small volumes of dexamethasone or a similar steroid, or mitomycin-C submucosally at the area of the stricture. Stenting may be required in cases of recurrent stenosis but mechanical dilation commonly requires serial procedures and most centers would utilize a multimodality approach and recommends dilation on at least two occasions prior to considering stent placement. Dilation allows for better evaluation of the extent of the stenosis and the airways distal to the narrowing. In addition if the stenosis is secondary to either infection or inflammation of the airway, serial dilations may allow improved airway function while the primary process (infection or rejection) is aggressively treated, which may improve the long term result and in many cases avoid stent placement. There is debate regarding the ideal stent for placement in stenotic airways. Silcone stents commonly require rigid bronchoscopy for placement. However they have several advantages including lower rates of granulation tissue, easy removal, ability to modify and customize (length and create customized holes for ventilation and secretion clearance). The disadvantage is that they are prone to problems with secretion clearance and plugging and migration. The advantage of self-expandable metallic stents is their ease of deployment using a flexible bronchoscope and flexibility, but they can also exacerbate the fibrosis and granulation response of the airway. They are also extremely difficult to remove once placed.

Segmental non-anastomotic bronchial stenosis or bronchomalacia (3 percent) can be seen in persons with infectious complications or in patients with multiple bouts of acute airway rejection. Treatment of the underlying infection or rejection is critical to managing these complications and may result in resolution of the stenosis. Alternatively mechanical balloon dilation and less commonly stent placement can be performed if the airway is proximal and large enough to allow successful placement.

Tracheobronchomalacia

Tracheobronchomalacia can occur in combination with bronchial stenosis or independently and is also commonly associated with cartilaginous injury due to perioperative ischemia, recurrent bronchial infection, and/or rejection. Inspiratory and expiratory CT scans can be diagnostic however direct visualization or the airway with flexible bronchoscopy is the gold standard for diagnosis to help guide decisions regarding management. While tracheo-bronchomalacia does not respond to balloon dilation, stent placement may improve airway patency. Silicone stents are preferred.

Granulation Tissue

Granulation tissue can form in response to prior injury or secondary to a foreign body reaction. The suture material can stimulate a granulation tissue response. If airway obstruction is present secondary to granulation tissue, several techniques for debridement are available including mechanical debridement using a forceps, cryotherapy, electrocautery, laser, and APC. Alternatively, local injection of corticosteroids has been used. The use of laser may cause thermal burns deep beneath the mucosal tissues and induce more scarring and granulation tissue formation or stenosis and should be used with caution. Recurrence is common and repeated therapy with a multimodality approach may be needed.

Anastomotic Dehiscence

Anastomotic dehiscence may be partial or complete. Complete dehiscence is very difficult to treat and associated with high mortality. Incomplete or partial dehiscence can be managed conservatively with frequent bronchoscopies to clear blood and necrotic tissue along with antibiotic therapy. In some cases temporary stenting, taking advantage of the propensity of metallic stents to cause granulation tissue, may stabilize the airway to allow healing. However stent placement should not be performed in the presence of an active infection. Endoscopic repair of an anastomotic dehiscence using injection of alpha-cyanoacrylate glue has also been reported. As surgical technique has improved, the incidence of dehiscence has been decreasing and this is a rare complication under current practice.

Bronchial Fistulae

Fistulas of the bronchial tree are rare but challenging complications. Three types have been reported; bronchomediastinal, bronchovascular, and bronchopleural. Bronchial ischemia and/or infection are felt to be a contributing factor in all the three types of fistulas. Management depends on the timing, size, and the patients overall condition. Flexible bronchoscopy can be helpful in localizing either a bronchomediastinal or bronchovascular fistula but endoscopic therapeutic options are limited, especially when infection is a contributing factor. Successful endoscopic techniques using fibrin or cyanoacrylate glue or placement of endobronchial valves have been reported for the treatment of bronchopleural fistulas.

Anastomotic Infections

Bacterial or fungal infections of the bronchial anastomosis are associated with poor healing of the anastomosis. Diagnosis of anastomotic infections is usually done using bronchoscopy and these infections are commonly polymicrobial. Treatment includes bronchoscopic debridement, which often requires serial procedures over long periods of time in combination with aggressive antimicrobial therapy to achieve adequate control. Long term sequelae including stenosis or bronchomalacia may occur that require dilation or stenting. However placement of a stent is not recommended acutely until the infection is under control or ideally totally resolved.

Learning Points:

1. Bronchoscopy is a pivotal procedure in the management of lung transplant patients.
2. There are four main indications for bronchoscopy following lung transplantation;

   a. Evaluation and management of the potential lung donor
   b. Surveillance bronchoscopy with TBBx for rejection
   c. Diagnostic bronchoscopy for changes in clinical status
   d. Visualization of the anastomosis and management of airway complications including airway debridement, dilation, and/or stent placement

3. The performance of bronchoscopy in the lung transplant patient is the same as for non-transplant patients, with the following exceptions;

   a. The immunocompromised status of the patients widens the differential of potential pathogens that may cause infectious complications
   b. The cough reflex is blunted in lung transplant patients, which influences the risk of silent aspiration but can also improve tolerance of the procedure.

4. Some reports suggest an increased risk of bleeding with TBBx independent of other known bleeding risks, but the procedure can be safely and effectively performed in this patient population.
5. There is debate among transplant centers regarding the utility of performing routine surveillance bronchoscopy with TBBx among lung transplant patients.

Further Readings

Burguete SR, Maselli DJ, Fernandez JF, Levine SM. Lung transplant infection. *Respirology*. 2013;18: 22–38.

Cooper JD, Patterson GA, Trulock EP. Results of single and bilateral lung transplantation in 131 consecutive recipients. Washington University Lung Transplant Group. *J Thorac Cardiovasc Surg*. 1994;107(2):460–470; discussion 470–471.

Courad L, Nashef SAM, Nicolini P, Jougon J. Classification of airway anastomotic healing. *Eur J Cardiothoracic Surg*. 1992;6:496–497.

DeVito Dabbs A, Hoffman LA, Iacono AT, et al. Are symptom reports useful for differentiating between acute rejection and pulmonary infection after lung transplantation? *Heart Lung*. 2004; 33(6):372–380.

Diette GB, Wiener CM, White P. The higher risk of bleeding in lung transplant recipients from bronchoscopy is independent of traditional bleeding risks: results of a prospective cohort study. *Chest*. 1999;115(2):397–402.

Dransfield MT, Garver RI, Weill D. Standardized guidelines for surveillance bronchoscopy to reduce complication in lung transplant recipients. *J Heart Lung Transplant*. 2004;23(1):110–114.

Dutau H, Vandemoortele T, Laroumagne S, Gomez C, Boussaud V, Cavailles A, Cellerin L, Colchen A, Degot T, Gonin F, Hermant C, Jougon J, Kessler R, Philit F, Pison C, Raymond CS, Wermert D, Astoul P, Thomas P, Reynaud-Gaubert M, Vergnon JM. A new endoscopic standardized grading system for macroscopic central airway complications following lung transplantation: the MDS classification. *European Journal of Cardio-Thoracic Surgery*. 2014;45:e33–e38.

Griffith BP, Zenati M. The pulmonary donor. *Clin Chest Med*. 1990;11(2):217–226.

Guilinger RA, Paradis IL, Dauber JH, et al. The importance of bronchoscopy with transbronchial biopsy and bronchoalveolar lavage in the management of lung transplant recipients. *Am J Respir Crit Care Med*. 1995;152(6 Pt 1):2037–2043.

Kukafka DS, O'Brien GM, Furukawa S, Criner GJ. Surveillance bronchoscopy in lung transplant recipients. *Chest*. 1997;111(2):377–381.

Levine SM. Transplant/Immunology Network of the American College of Chest Physicians. A survey of clinical practice of lung transplantation in North America. *Chest*. 2004;125(4):1224–1238.

Machuzak M, Santacruz JF, Gildea T, Murthy SC. Airway complications after lung transplantation. *Thorac Surg Clin*. 2015;25:55–75.

Orens JB, Estenne M, Arcasoy S, et al. Pulmonary Scientific Council of the International Society for Heart and Lung Transplantation. International guidelines for the selection of lung transplant candidates: 2006 update–a consensus report from the Pulmonary Scientific Council of the International Society for Heart and Lung Transplantation. *J Heart Lung Transplant*. 2006;25(7): 745–755.

Pomerance A, Madden B, Buke MM, Yacoub MH. Transbronchial biopsy in heart and lung transplantation: clinicopathologic correlations. *J Heart Lung Transplant*. 1995;14(4):761–773.

Riou B, Guesde R, Jacquens Y, Duranteau R, Viars P. Fiberoptic bronchoscopy in brain-dead organ donors. *Am J Respir Crit Care Med*. 1994;150(2):558–560.

Shennib H, Massard G. Airway complications in lung transplantation. *Ann Thorac Surg*. 1994;57: 506–551.

Stewart S, Fishbein MC, Snell GI, Berry GJ, Boehler A, Burke MM, Glanville A, Gould FK, Magro C, Marboe CC, McNeil KD, Reed EF, Reinsmoen NL, Scott JP, Studer SM, Tazelaar HD, Wallwork JL, Westall G, Zamora MR, Zeevi A, Yousem SA. Revision of the 1996 Working Formulation for the Standardization of Nomenclature in the Diagnosis of Lung Rejection. *J Heart Lung Transplant*. 2007;26:1229–1242.

Tiroke AH, Bewig B, Haverich A. Bronchoalveolar lavage in lung transplantation. State of the art. *Clin Transplant*. 1999;13(2):131–157.

Trulock EP, Ettinger NA, Brunt EM, Pasque MK, Kaiser LR, Cooper JD. The role of transbronchial lung biopsy in the treatment of lung transplant recipients. An analysis of 200 consecutive procedures. *Chest*. 1992;102(4):1049–1054.

Valentine VG, Taylor DE, Dhillon GS, et al. Success of lung transplantation without surveillance bronchoscopy. *J Heart Lung Transplant*. 2002;21(3):319–326.

Wahidi MM, Ernst A. The role of bronchoscopy in the management of lung transplant recipients. *Respir Care Clin*. 2004;10:549–562.

Yousem SA. Significance of clinically silent untreated mild acute cellular rejection in lung allograft recipients. *Hum Pathol*. 1996;27(3):269–273.

Yousem SA, Paradis I, Griffith BP. Can transbronchial biopsy aid in the diagnosis of bronchiolitis obliterans in lung transplant recipients? *Transplantation*. 1994;57(1):151–153.

Chapter 15

Basic Navigational Bronchoscopy

Dominik Harzheim and Jonas Herth

A solitary pulmonary nodule (SPN) is a round or oval opacity smaller than 3 cm in diameter that is completely surrounded by pulmonary parenchyma. Owing to the high etiological diversity and the potential for malignancy, pulmonary nodules represent a clinical challenge, which becomes increasingly frequent as the number of CT examinations rises. Due to its low sensitivity, a bronchoscopic approach to small pulmonary nodules <2 cm in diameter was previously not recommended by *The American College of Chest Physicians*. With the recent advent of innovative guidance technics for bronchoscopic sampling, this statement was revised, taking the higher diagnostic yield of navigation systems such as endobronchial ultrasound, guide sheath, virtual bronchoscopy, and electromagnetic navigation into account. By means of these methods, the identification of malignant nodules measuring ≤ 2 cm could be raised from a prior reported overall sensitivity of 33 percent for fluoroscopy-guided bronchoscopy with transbronchial biopsy (TBB) to a pooled diagnostic yield of 61 percent.

The following chapter will give an overview of the different earlier mentioned navigation technics.

Endobronchial Ultrasound for Peripheral Lesions

In the diagnosis of peripheral lung lesions, radial probe endobronchial ultrasound (EBUS) provides real-time confirmation of the target lesion localization. This method currently depicts the most practically used bronchoscopic device in the diagnosis of peripheral lung lesions. Consisting of a rotating piezoelectric crystal embedded in a flexible catheter, the miniaturized transducer, also referred to as miniprobe, produces a 360° ultrasound image. The most commonly used frequency of the EBUS probe is 20 MHz which allowes for a high resolution of <1 mm and a penetration depth of around 4 cm. Aside from the excellent depiction of the airway wall with its different layers, it enables the investigation of peribronchial structures not only within the mediastinum, but also in the lung periphery. For the purpose of diagnosing peripheral lung lesions and pulmonary nodules, the miniprobe is advanced into different bronchi like a forceps. Unlike the forceps, the EBUS probe must be handled carefully due to its fragility. Based on the pre-procedure CT scan, the miniprobe is inserted into the segmental bronchi where the lesion is suspected. In case the operator perceives a high resistance while introducing the probe deeper into the desired bronchus, one can dilate the airway through prior insertion of a sampling forceps. By this means damage to the transducer or the connecting drive wire by shear forces and flexion can be prevented.

While advancing the miniprobe through the airway, a characteristic "snowstormlike" whitish ultrasound image (Figure 15.1), produced by air-filled alveolar tissue, can be seen. Due to the total reflection of ultrasound waves by air, structures that are close to the probe but separated by air cannot be inspected. Particularly in the proximal airways, vessels, appearing

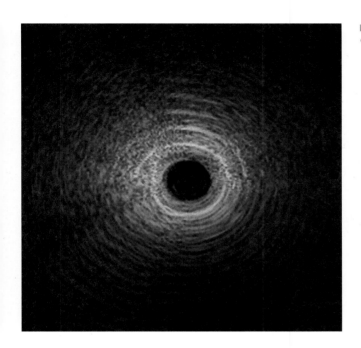

Figure 15.1 Typical EBUS image of normal peripheral lung.

totally black, are often noticed. Owing to the lack of color doppler imaging in radial EBUS imaging, it is sometimes difficult to clearly differentiate between vessels and necrotic areas. By tracking the structure in its entirety and looking for potential arterial pulsation it is usually possible to make a clear differentiation. Once a solid tumor is reached, the ultrasound image will change to a homogeneous grey ultrasound image with plain white borders indicating the borders of the lesion (Figure 15.2). Continuous hyper echoic margins and the absence of an air bronchogram further raise the suspicion for cancer. Dark inhomogeneous zones however, do not exclude malignancy since necrotic areas and vessels within the tumor might be visible. Atelectasis or inflammatory tissue is characterized by an inhomogeneous image resulting from different structures like fluid filled dark structures and sharp white echoes from small bronchi without plain borders (Figure 15.3).

Once having localized the target lesion, a methodological limitation of the EBUS-TBB approach constitutes the removal of the ultrasonic probe from the bronchoscope prior to the introduction of biopsy instruments. The procedure is not "real-time"; hence, the detection of the identic subsegmental bronchus after removal of the miniprobe can be problematic. This is often aggravated by the different rigidity of the bronchoscope after insertion of the biopsy forceps into the working channel. Furthermore, due to its higher rigidity, the biopsy forceps sometimes takes another path in the distal bronchial distribution as the miniprobe.

To overcome this constraint, the operator has mainly two options. First introduced by Kurimoto, the endobronchial ultrasound can be used in combination with a *guide sheath*. For the 1.4-mm measuring miniprobes, catheters with a diameter of 2.0 mm can be used, whereas the larger 1.7-mm probes should be employed with catheters of a 2.7-mm diameter. The probe is advanced through the guide sheath which serves as an extended working channel. Once the lesion is reached and confirmed via EBUS, the miniprobe is extracted while the guide sheath is kept in place. Now different biopsy instruments can be

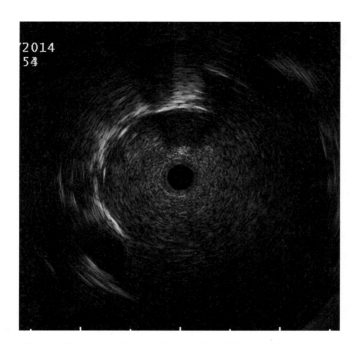

Figure 15.2 EBUS image of a solitary pulmonary nodule.

advanced through the guide sheath which enables sampling at the exact same position as the miniprobe before. If the target bronchus cannot be intubated due to the required angle, a double-hinged curette can be used in order to lead the guide sheath in successfully reaching the lesion. Before usage, the miniprobe has to be removed from the guide sheath in order to

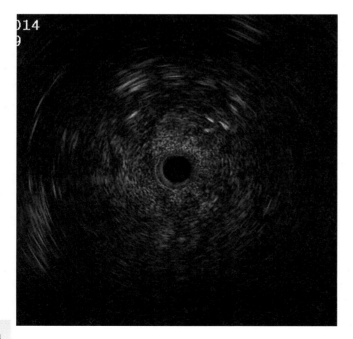

Figure 15.3 EBUS image of an or inflammatory process (inhomogeneous image, resulting from different structures like fluid filled dark structures and sharp white echoes)

allow the double-hinged curette to be inserted. Once the desired bronchus is reached under fluoroscopic guidance, the miniprobe can be reinstalled.

Another EBUS guiding option is the *fluoroscopic* registration of the miniprobe position once the target lesion is reached. By means of intermittent fluoroscopic guidance, the biopsy tool can be advanced to the identical location as the prior miniprobe. A potential benefit of this approach is the shorter duration and retrenchment at expense of radiation burden. Since fluoroscopic and EBUS guidance are frequently combined in order to reach the target lesion, the fluoroscopic registration of the miniprobe seldom depicts an extra effort.

Particularly in case of small pulmonary nodules, which can seldom be visualized by fluoroscopy, EBUS guidance offers an advantage. A prospective study investigating the diagnostic yield of EBUS in fluoroscopically invisible lung lesions could establish a diagnosis by biopsy in 70 percent of the cases. In pulmonary nodules <2 cm, a diagnostic yield of 69 percent was reported if the lesion could be visualized by EBUS. Another study could show the usefulness of EBUS guidance in combination with guide sheath as a stand-alone guidance technic. A systematic review of published literature evaluating radial probe EBUS accuracy showed a sensitivity (73 percent) and specificity (100 percent) markedly higher than for routine bronchoscopy. However a significant inter-study variation in EBUS method was noted.

Virtual Bronchoscopic Navigation / Ultrathin Bronchoscopy

Virtual Bronchoscopy (VB) is a relative novel technique for the noninvasive evaluation of the tracheobronchial tree. Through reconstruction of helical CT images it creates a three-dimensional rendering resembling the bronchoscopical investigation of the lung. Except radiation exposure, VB has no adverse effects but requires thin-section CT scans with a slice thickness of 1.25 mm or less, depending on the system used. The level of anatomic detail visualized by VB depends on the obtained volume data. In general, good volume data are obtained by minimizing collimation and overlapping the image reconstruction by at least 50 percent.

Until recently VB has been used mainly for the investigation of trachea and bronchi in children, evaluation of airway stenosis, endobronchial malignancy, postoperative bronchial complications, and the study of anatomic malformation and variants.

Prior to a bronchoscopical investigation of a pulmonary nodule, the bronchoscopist aims to determine the bronchial path leading to the desired target based on CT images. However, it can be difficult to obtain a three-dimensional understanding of the complicated tracheobronchial tree solely relying on axial images. By providing a three-dimensional depiction of the bronchial path to the lesion, VB resolves this problem. Particularly for the usage of ultrathin bronchoscopes with external diameters of 3 cm, this might be a key advantage. Whereas standard bronchoscopes are limited to the first three to four divisions of the bronchial tree, ultrathin bronchoscopes can be advanced to a median of the sixth generation bronchi. Here VBN comes into play since guidance in the deeper bronchial tree gets more difficult with every branching. In case of successful guidance, subsequent sampling by forceps is easier due to the closer advance of the ultrathin bronchoscope to the pulmonary nodule. In addition, the ultrathin bronchoscope can be advanced to lesions in places such as the mediastinal side of the lung apex that are difficult to reach with a conventional bronchoscope.

Current VBN guidance systems include, but are not limited to the LungPoint System by Broncus Technologies and the VBN system Bf-NAVI by Olympus Medical Systems. Those Systems process recorded CT data in order to automatically compile three-dimensional VB

175

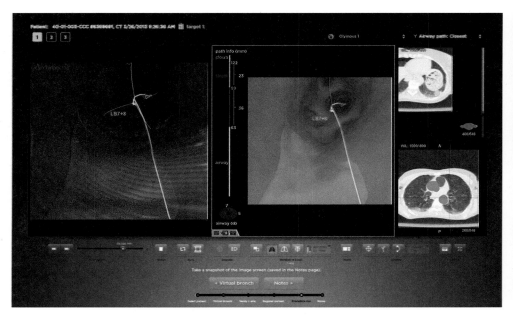

Figure 15.4 Virtual track of the LungPoint system in the CT navigation image (left) and in the real time image (right)

images. Once the operator chooses the target, up to three pathways are calculated to reach this point closest as possible. A virtual bronchoscopic animation enables the estimation of the calculated pathways prior to the intervention. During the intervention, VB images are synchronized with real images for bronchoscopic navigation (Figure 15.4). Since the tip of the bronchoscope can only be steered in one axis, variable rotation of the scope is necessary at every bronchus branching. This causes a shift of the virtual and real image to a greater or lesser extent. To overcome this issue, an assistant adjusts the virtual images produced by the Bf-NAVI system by using the forward, backward, and rotation function. As the bronchial branching pattern includes many bifurcations into two bronchi of similar sizes, mistakes tend to be made identifying the bronchus into which the bronchoscope should be advanced. Therefore, careful alignment of the virtual and real image is necessary prior to further bronchoscope advancement. After reconciliation, VB images of the next branching indicate the proper path for the subsequent bronchoscope advancement. This procedure is repeated until the target bronchus is reached. As a result of unexpected patient movements such as coughing, a substantial image shift might emerge. In this case, VB images can be redisplayed and thumbnails of each branching provide a reference.

The LungPoint system offers a slightly different solution for the earlier-discussed issues of image shifting and unexpected patient movement. The system displays VB image and the bronchoscopic video next to each other and overlays the correct path to the target airway on both images in blue. An image-based synchronization technique aligns virtual image and bronchus anatomy seen through the bronchoscope. This process can be accelerated or corrected by an assistant by advancement and adjustment of the virtual bronchoscopic rendering. The system not only displays airways measuring 3 mm and greater, but also extracts major vessels. Those and the target can be overlaid on the VB image to further facilitate navigation and increase procedure safety.

One study evaluating the LungPoint system showed a mean planning time of five minutes and a mean examination time of 15 minutes. In general, VBN seems to reduce the bronchoscopic examination time by facilitating its navigation. This holds true especially for procedures applying an ultrathin bronchoscope.

VBN studies available to date show a high diagnostic yield of 73 percent by sampling 428 lesions with a slightly lower yield of 67 percent for lesions <2 cm. However, concerning the usefulness of combining ultrathin bronchoscopes and VBN, conflicting evidence exists. This might be owed to the possibility that VBN is more useful for non-expert bronchoscopists, since highly trained operators might be able to assume the route to the desired target to some extent from CT images alone.

One limitation of ultrathin bronchoscopes depicts the restriction to miniaturized sampling tools and therefore the extraction of merely small tissue samples. In future, this might be overcome by small cryoprobes designed for tissue sampling through ultrathin bronchoscopes.

Electromagnetic Navigation

In contrast to VBN, electromagnetic navigation bronchoscopy (ENB) depicts a real-time procedure with the ability of mapping instruments within an electromagnetic field. It resembles a GPS car system whereby the operator knows the position of the instruments at any point of the procedure. Examples for ENB are the Superdimension and the Veran guidance system. ENB not only provides guiding to peripheral lung lesions but also to mediastinal and hilar lymph nodes.

Similar to VBN, ENB requires high-quality CT scans in order to provide adequate resolution for the creation of a 3D map of the airways. In case of the Superdimension system, cuts of 1.5 mm or less and a 1.0 mm overlap are necessary. The Superdimension system is composed of four main components: a disposable working channel and guide catheter, a software which provides the physician with planning and navigation views of the lungs via merged CT images and hardware including computer, monitors, and an electromagnetic location board. The location board emits low-frequency electromagnetic waves during the procedure and is placed under the cranial end of the mattress on the bronchoscopy table.

After CT image registration by the ENB software, the operator can determine several targets to which navigation is desired. The software then suggests a pathway to the chosen target and provides a 3D film of the appropriate route. It can be adjusted as deemed necessary.

In the following registration phase the patient lies down on the location board and three sensors are placed on the body, serving as markers for the system.

Subsequently, electromagnetic guidance is achieved through a sensor incorporated in the distal tip of a steerable navigation catheter. It can be tracked by means of the electromagnetic field created by the locator board and matched to the information contained in the CT scan analyzed in the planning phase. Together with the extended working channel the navigation catheter is inserted into the bronchoscopes working channel. Once the bronchoscope cannot proceed any more, the steerable guide catheter is advanced by turning and pulling the control lever on the catheter's handle. The first version of the catheter was steered by four separate wires controlling the movement of the probe from the proximal end of the device thus allowing its distal section to be steered in a complete circle (360°). The location and steering

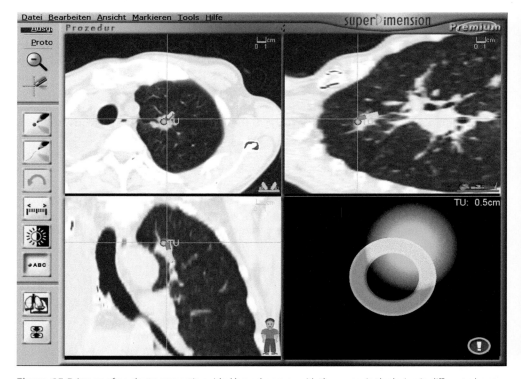

Figure 15.5 Image of an electromagnetic guided bronchoscopy with the sensor in the lesion in different planes.

directions are performed according to the sensors' position on the CT roadmap leading to the target that was previously registered to the patient's lung. When reaching an airway bifurcation, the catheter is steered by manipulating the handle. A triangle depicted on the handles dial indicates the direction of the catheters tip. By pulling the handle, the tip is brought into the desired position. After reaching the target, the extended working channel is kept into place whereas the navigation catheter is removed. The extended working channel now serves as an extension of the bronchoscopes channel similar to a guide sheath. Tissue sampling can now be performed. A recently introduced, updated version of the steerable guide catheter has a curved tip. Through this, it can be steered more easily by simply rotating the catheters handle (Figure 15.5).

One study reported on the influence the adjustment of CT scan and patient has on diagnostic yield. In case of a discrepancy <4.4 mm, the diagnostic yield was 71 percent, whereas it dropped to 40 percent where discrepancies were >4.4 mm. While the size of lesions had no significant impact on diagnostic yield, sampling in the lower lobes showed a lower yield. This might be due to a higher navigation error occurring in more peripheral lesions. This also applies to lesions near the diaphragm caused by permanent movement within the respiratory cycle. These drawbacks might be overcome to some degree by the recently implemented automatic registration of the system.

A recent meta-analysis characterized ENB to be effective and safe. It showed an overall sensitivity of 71 percent in the detection of cancer by sampling 1033 nodules.

The major challenge to ENB depicts the high costs of the procedure. In case of the SuperDimension system, the single use locatable guide costs between US $700 and $1000, depending on the market.

Conclusion

In recent years, bronchoscopic navigation technics have led to a distinct improvement in the diagnosis of peripheral lung lesions without compromising safety. Hereby, bronchoscopy nowadays competes with the transthoracic approach to small lung lesions. While EBUS already depicts a frequently used technic, commonly available in many bronchoscopic suits, VB and EMN yet remain rarely employed navigation tools. First, this is due to high costs involved and second, it is due to concomitant technologic requirements.

In order to further raise the diagnostic yield, navigation technics have yet been successfully combined. By this means, the combination of EBUS with EMN or VB have shown to overcome each individual technic's limitation.

Owing to the high accuracy of new navigation technics, bronchoscopic treatment of lung cancer might play an increasing part in near future. Placement of fiducial markers for stereotactic radiosurgery, endoluminal brachytherapy, and minimally invasive radiotherapy yet depict feasible technics. Radiofrequency ablation probes for the endoscopic treatment of small lung lesions in non-surgical patients are in development and might become a competing approach to transthoracic percutaneous radiofrequency ablation.

Further Readings

Asano F. Virtual bronchoscopic navigation. *Clin Chest Med.* 2010 Mar;31(1):75–85.

Asano F, Shinagawa N, Ishida T, Shindoh J, Anzai M, Tsuzuku A, et al. Virtual bronchoscopic navigation combined with ultrathin bronchoscopy. *A Randomized Clinical Trial. Am J Respir Crit Care Med.* 2013 Aug;188(3):327–333.

Eberhardt R, Ernst A, Herth FJF. Ultrasound-guided transbronchial biopsy of solitary pulmonary nodules less than 20 mm. *Eur Respir J.* 2009 Dec;34(6):1284–1287.

Eberhardt R, Anantham D, Ernst A, Feller-Kopman D, Herth F. Multimodality bronchoscopic diagnosis of peripheral lung lesions. *Am J Respir Crit Care Med.* 2007 Jul 1;176(1):36–41.

Eberhardt R, Kahn N, Gompelmann D, Schumann M, Heussel CP, Herth FJF. LungPoint–a new approach to peripheral lesions. *J Thorac Oncol Off Publ Int Assoc Study Lung Cancer.* 2010 Oct; 5(10):1559–1563.

Gex G, Pralong JA, Combescure C, Seijo L, Rochat T, Soccal PM. Diagnostic yield and safety of electromagnetic navigation bronchoscopy for lung nodules: a systematic review and meta-analysis. *Respir Int Rev Thorac Dis.* 2014;87(2):165–176.

Gould MK, Donington J, Lynch WR, Mazzone PJ, Midthun DE, Naidich DP, et al. Evaluation of individuals with pulmonary nodules: when is it lung cancer? Diagnosis and management of lung cancer, 3rd ed: American College of Chest Physicians evidence-based clinical practice guidelines. *Chest.* 2013 May;143(5 Suppl):e93S–120S.

Herth FJF, Eberhardt R, Becker HD, Ernst A. Endobronchial ultrasound-guided transbronchial lung biopsy in fluoroscopically invisible solitary pulmonary nodules*: A prospective trial. *Chest.* 2006 Jan 1;129(1):147–50.

Ishida T, Asano F, Yamazaki K, Shinagawa N, Oizumi S, Moriya H, et al. Virtual bronchoscopic navigation combined with endobronchial ultrasound to diagnose small peripheral pulmonary lesions: a randomised trial. *Thorax.* 2011 Dec;66(12):1072–1077.

Kanemoto K, Satoh H, Ishikawa H, Kagohashi K, Kurishima K, Sekizawa K. Diagnostic procedures for small pulmonary nodules detected by mass-screening. *Anticancer Res.* 2008 Oct;28(5B): 3153–3155.

Kurimoto N, Miyazawa T, Okimasa S, Maeda A, Oiwa H, Miyazu Y, et al. Endobronchial ultrasonography using a guide sheath increases the ability to diagnose peripheral pulmonary lesions endoscopically. *Chest.* 2004 Sep;126(3):959–965.

Neumann K, Winterer J, Kimmig M, Burger D, Einert A, Allmann K-H, et al. Real-time interactive virtual endoscopy of the tracheo–bronchial system: influence of CT imaging protocols and observer ability. *Eur J Radiol.* 2000 Jan;33(1):50–54.

Rivera MP, Mehta AC. Initial diagnosis of lung cancer: ACCP evidence-based clinical practice guidelines (2nd edition). *CHEST J.* 2007 Sep 1;132(3 suppl):131S–148S.

Schreiber G, McCrory DC. Performance characteristics of different modalities for diagnosis of suspected lung cancer*: Summary of published evidence. *CHEST J.* 2003 Jan 1;123(1 suppl): 115S–128S.

Schuhmann M, Bostanci K, Bugalho A, Warth A, Schnabel PA, Herth FJF, et al. Endobronchial ultrasound-guided cryobiopsies in peripheral pulmonary lesions: a feasibility study. *Eur Respir J.* 2014 Jan;43(1):233–239.

Schwarz Y, Greif J, Becker HD, Ernst A, Mehta A. Real-time electromagnetic navigation bronchoscopy to peripheral lung lesions using overlaid CT images: The first human study. *Chest.* 2006 Apr 1;129(4):988–994.

Tanabe T, Koizumi T, Tsushima K, Ito M, Kanda S, Kobayashi T, et al. Comparative study of three different catheters for CT imaging-bronchoscopy-guided radiofrequency ablation as a potential and novel interventional therapy for lung cancer. *Chest.* 2010 Apr;137(4):890–897.

Wang Memoli JS, Nietert PJ, Silvestri GA. Meta-analysis of Guided Bronchoscopy for the Evaluation of the Pulmonary Nodule. *Chest.* 2012 Aug;142(2):385–393.

Yoshikawa M, Sukoh N, Yamazaki K, Kanazawa K, Fukumoto S, Harada M, et al. Diagnostic value of endobronchial ultrasonography with a guide sheath for peripheral pulmonary lesions without X-ray fluoroscopy. *Chest.* 2007 Jun;131(6):1788–1793.

Chapter 16

Basic Therapeutic Techniques

Luis F. Angel and Deborah J. Levine

Introduction

Interventional pulmonology is an evolving discipline stemming from pulmonary medicine that concentrates on both diagnostic and therapeutic interventions for patients with advanced airway and pleural diseases. The interventional pulmonologist has taken an active role in developing potentially less invasive ways to perform diagnostic and therapeutic procedures in disorders of the airway and pleura.

Procedures encompassed within this expanding field include, but are not limited to, rigid bronchoscopy, endobronchial laser therapy, electrocautery, cryotherapy, balloon dilation (BD), brachytherapy (BT), and endotracheal or endobronchial stent placement. The question of which modality to use is influenced by many factors, including patient presentation, operator proficiency, anesthetic techniques, and the institution's available equipment. The key to success in caring for patients with these disorders is careful patient selection and the complementary application of these techniques. In this review we will focus on describing these procedures, as well as outlining an active approach to the clinical disorders for which they are used.

Central Airways Obstruction

Obstruction or stenosis of the trachea and large bronchi can be a consequence of endobronchial obstruction, extraluminal compression, or a combination of both. Endoluminal or endobronchial lesions are most common. Extrinsic compression causing obstruction of the airway is less frequent, but can result in symptoms and outcomes similar to those of endobronchial obstruction. Most cases are secondary to bronchogenic carcinoma; however, both benign and malignant causes can produce significant morbidity and decreased life expectancy if left untreated. Table 16.1 shows the common etiologies of central airway obstruction.

The presenting symptoms of airway obstruction will differ depending on the anatomic location and severity of the obstruction. Symptoms range from chronic hoarseness, cough, dyspnea, and wheezing to more severe acute problems such as stridor, hemoptysis, and respiratory failure. When approaching the patient with upper airway obstruction, the pulmonologist must take into account the stability of the patient, the underlying pathologic condition, and the short-and long-term prognoses of the disease process. The location and severity of the lesion and the rate of progression of the obstruction are significant aspects that need to be considered when evaluating these difficult conditions. The availability of equipment and the expertise of the interventionalist are also important factors in deciding how to treat the

Table 16.1 Conditions Associated with Central Airway Obstruction

Malignant	Nonmalignant
Primary endoluminal carcinoma:	Lymphadenopathy:
Bronchogenic	Sarcoidosis
Adenoid cystic	Infectious (i.e., tuberculosis)
Mucoepidermoid	Vascular:
Carcinoid	Sling
Metastatic carcinoma to the airway:	Cartilage:
Bronchogenic	Relapsing polychondritis
Renal cell	Granulation tissue from:
Breast	Endotracheal tubes
Thyroid	Tracheostomy tubes
Colon	Airway stents
Sarcoma	Foreign bodies
Melanoma	Surgical anastomoses
Laryngeal carcinoma	Wegener's granulomatosis
Esophageal carcinoma	Pseudotumor:
Mediastinal tumors:	Hamartomas
Thymus	Amyloid
Thyroid	Papillomatosis
Germ cell	Hyperdynamic:
Lymphadenopathy associated with any of the above malignancies:	Tracheomalacia
	Bronchomalacia
Lymphoma	Other:
	Goiter
	Mucus plug
	Vocal cord paralysis
	Epiglottitis
	Blood clot

individual patient. Most patients will require a combination of various techniques for the most successful outcomes.

Rigid Bronchoscopy

The rigid bronchoscope is an invaluable tool that allows the interventional pulmonologist to secure, evaluate, and manipulate the trachea and proximal bronchi, while controlling oxygenation and ventilation. It is the most rapid technique to relieve an obstruction of the central airways, whether it is an intraluminal or extraluminal obstruction.

Today, a majority of bronchoscopies are being performed with the flexible scope; making it the procedure of choice for most diagnostic and some therapeutic procedures. Despite this rapid expansion and widespread use of the flexible scope, however, the rigid scope still

Table 16.2 Comparison of Rigid and Flexible Bronchoscopy

	Rigid Bronchoscopy	Flexible Bronchoscopy
Expertise	7 percent of practicing pulmonologists	95 percent of practicing pulmonologists
Anesthesia	General anesthesia	Conscious sedation
Oxygenation and ventilation	Excellent support for both with jet or conventional ventilation	Poor support for oxygenation and ventilation
Bleeding control	Better visualization and suctioning	Poor visualization and ineffective suction
Location of the lesion	Ideal for central and large airways lesions	Easy access to central and distal airways
Size of biopsies	Large	Small
Mechanical debridement	More effective and efficient	Less effective and time consuming
Foreign body removal	Easier and effective in large or central airways	Effective but may be more difficult and time consuming
Management of critical airway narrowing	Gold standard	May worsen airway obstruction
Dilatation of strictures	Mechanical dilation possible with the rigid scope	Possible with the use of balloon dilation

remains an imperative tool for therapeutic practice. Both flexible and rigid bronchoscopy have unique characteristics and offer specific advantages depending on the clinical situation. Table 16.2 compares rigid and flexible bronchoscopy and the best indications for specific clinical scenarios.

For patients with respiratory insufficiency secondary to central airways obstruction, reestablishment of the airway can be accomplished with intubation and advancement of the rigid scope. The airway can then be dilated by the advancement of the scope along the wall of the airway. This dilation may be temporary, but will allow oxygenation, ventilation, and time to evaluate the obstructed area for further therapy. If the airway is too narrow to allow advancement of the scope, balloons of increasing diameter can be passed through the scope for dilation. The scope can then be used as a tumor-debulking instrument, by "corkscrewing" the scope to core out large pieces of tumor. In patients with extrinsic compression causing airway obstruction, the rigid bronchoscope is required for the insertion of silicone stents in the trachea or proximal bronchi. Rigid bronchoscopy is also a vital tool in controlling massive hemoptysis. Hemorrhage can be controlled by tamponade with the scope and with the use of large suction catheters to remove blood or clots.

With proper technique and safe anesthesia, there are few complications associated with rigid bronchoscopy. The most common problems come during intubation or advancement of the scope, causing trauma to the teeth, oropharynx, trachea, or bronchial walls. Massive bleeding is rare. There are few contraindications to rigid bronchoscopy, and most are related to use of general anesthesia. These include unstable cardiopulmonary status and serious arrhythmias.

Laser

Laser therapy is a recognized endobronchial treatment that the interventional pulmonologist uses today. It is used extensively for the palliation of symptoms of airway obstruction secondary to malignancies, and it provides effective therapy for benign airway lesions and stenosis. In selected patients, laser therapy has been shown to improve quality of life and functional status, and, in some cases, to extend survival.

The most widely used laser in the tracheobronchial tree is the neodymium-doped yttrium aluminium garnet (Nd:YAG) laser because of its deep penetration into tissues ($\leq$5 mm), superior coagulation characteristics, cutting ability, and versatility. It can be used through a flexible or rigid bronchoscope. The decision between using a flexible or rigid bronchoscope depends on the operator's experience, the character of the lesion, and patient stability. Lesions that are favorable to laser therapy include tracheal and main stem lesions, polypoid lesions of short length ($<$ 4 cm), lesions with a visible distal airway lumen, and functional lung distal to the obstruction. Lesions that are not favorable for laser resection have more than 80 percent obstruction of the airway and are those that destroy airway wall integrity and obliterate anatomical boundaries.

Palliation of symptoms from malignant airway obstruction is the most common indication for endobronchial laser therapy. It is also used for obstruction secondary to benign tumors such as hamartomas, papillomas, amyloidomas, and endobronchial endometriosis.

Bronchoscopic laser therapy is a relatively safe procedure. Most complications can be avoided by applying preventative safety measures. Perforation of a vascular structure, mediastinum, or esophagus is one of the most feared complications of laser therapy. Knowing the anatomic proximity of the aortic arch, pulmonary artery, and the esophagus is crucial when performing laser therapy near these areas. Another concerning complication is a laser-related endobronchial fire. Fires are uncommon when the rigid bronchoscope is used. Materials that ignite during laser therapy include the flexible scope sheath, endotracheal tubes, and silicone stents.

Contraindications to endobronchial laser therapy include extrinsic compression of the airway without an endobronchial lesion, involvement or compression of the pulmonary artery by tumor, tracheoesophageal fistula, and prolonged atelectasis for more than four weeks.

Electrocautery and Argon Plasma Coagulation

Although the Nd:YAG laser is recognized as the most widely used form of bronchoscopic intervention, its use may be limited by its expense, its relative lack of accessibility, and the belief that rigid bronchoscopy is required for its use. These factors have increased the appeal of a parallel procedure, electrocautery, which may be more available, more user friendly, and less expensive. Furthermore, there are many studies that present evidence that electrocautery has efficacy similar to that of laser therapy.

Bronchoscopic electrocautery, also called electrocoagulation (EC), unlike laser therapy, is usually performed in the contact mode, with the probe gently touching the tissue. A snare is available for polypoid lesions, and a standard probe is available for the bulky lesions. The indications, patient selection, and principles of application are essentially the same as for the Nd:YAG laser. Both benign and malignant lesions have proven to be amenable to electrocautery.

Complications are relatively similar to those of laser therapy, with hemorrhage, airway perforation, and (rarely) endobronchial fire. The EC probe needs to be cleaned from debris intermittently during the procedure, which is one disadvantage when comparing it with laser therapy. In general, however, EC has significant potential as an effective and cost-effective procedure for patients with endobronchial obstruction.

Argon plasma coagulation (APC) is a newer form of EC. It is used for both malignant and benign airway obstruction and endobronchial hemoptysis. It is used in the noncontact mode, similar to laser therapy. APC has the unique advantage of being able to treat lesions lateral to the probe. APC is less efficient than laser therapy at debulking large masses because it cannot generate as high of temperatures and provide as deep of tissue penetration.

Cryotherapy

Cryotherapy refers to the use of extreme cold for medical therapy. The goal of cryotherapy is to destroy pathologic tissue, while preserving normal mucosa. The basis of action relies on destruction of tissue by repeated cycles of freezing and thawing. Nitrous oxide (N_2O) is the most common cryogen used in endobronchial therapy.

There are many factors that influence tissue injury when cryotherapy is used. The absolute temperature, the rate of cooling and thawing, and the length of freezing time all affect the success of therapy. Freezing to $-40\,°C$ at the rate of $-100\,°C/min$ has been shown to cause >90 percent cell death. Tissue vascularity, the distance of tissue from the probe, the amount of water in the tissue, and the number of freeze–thaw cycles have also been found to be essential factors in the effectiveness of the therapy. The destruction of tissue by freezing occurs by both an immediate and delayed mechanism.

Tissues are either cryosensitive or cryoresistant, which is why certain tissues respond better than others to cryotherapy. Skin, mucous membranes, and granulation tissue (which arises histologically from mucous membranes) are cryosensitive, whereas fat cartilage and fibrous and connective tissue are cryoresistant. Tumor cells have been found to be more cryosensitive than are normal cells, making cryotherapy an attractive therapy for endobronchial malignancies.

The indications for cryotherapy are similar to those for laser and EC; however, each type of therapy has unique properties that may make one indicated over another in specific cases. Cryotherapy has been used most often for local therapy in the palliation of airway malignancies, and is also successfully used in benign airway conditions. It is effective in treating airway stenosis caused by excessive granulation tissue after lung transplant, and was reported to decrease the percentage of patients who required stent placement. Cryotherapy is excellent for papillomas as they are quite cryosensitive. It is successful in removing foreign bodies from the airway, especially objects that are friable or tend to fall apart with forceps. The object is frozen and then removed from the patient's airway with the probe and scope as one unit. This technique can also be used when removing blood clots and mucous plugs. Cryotherapy can decrease the risk of hemorrhage if performed prior to the biopsy of a suspected carcinoid lesion.

The lesions best treated with cryotherapy (whether they are benign or malignant) tend to be polypoid in nature and short in length, and they have a large endobronchial component. Long tapering lesions, bulky endobronchial lesions, or those with extensive submucosal involvement are not as favorable. Cryotherapy offers no benefit to patients with obstruction from pure extrinsic compression of the airway.

The advantages of cryotherapy are that it is a procedure that is easy to learn, relatively inexpensive (as compared with laser therapy), and safe. In comparison with laser or electrocautery, it does not have the danger of causing endobronchial fire. It is superior to modalities for distal lesions, as the risk of airway perforation is much lower. The cryoresistance of the bronchial tissue surrounding the lesions explains the safety of using cryotherapy. The main disadvantage of cryotherapy is that its effects are not immediate. It can take up to 2–4 weeks to show its maximum benefit and usually requires repeated bronchoscopies for follow-up and retreatment.

Balloon Dilation

In the past, non-emergent cases of airway stenosis have been treated by introducing rigid bronchoscopes of increasing diameters or by dilation by semirigid dilator. These techniques have been largely replaced by the use of BD performed using either rigid or flexible bronchoscopy. BD is an effective procedure to restore patency of airways that are narrowed from either benign or malignant processes. The great benefit of BD is that it is a relatively nontraumatic and rapid procedure to use in airway strictures. It is most frequently used in combination with other endobronchial techniques, but may be used alone in selected cases.

The balloon catheter is passed through the working channel of the bronchoscope or threaded over a guide wire (using the Seldinger method) and placed across the stenosis, with the balloon protruding slightly beyond either end. The balloon, which is slightly larger than the stenotic area, is then gradually inflated with water for 30–120 seconds at increasing pressures. Fluoroscopy has traditionally been used to monitor the inflation, but has been shown to be unnecessary when the stenotic region is visualized bronchoscopically. Serial dilations are performed with the same balloon or with one of a larger diameter until the airway lumen is restored. It is best to be able to visualize the airway distal to the stenosis to assess which size balloon should be used. This therapy has been shown to be best suited for stenotic areas that are short in length. Patients with transmural strictures that occupy a long segment of the airway usually require either surgical or stent therapy.

The major disadvantage of BD is that, although it can immediately dilate both intrinsic and extrinsic lesions, the results are usually not sustainable. Complications are rare, but include chest pain during inflation, bronchospasm, or atelectasis. Other possible complications include airway rupture or laceration by excessive balloon inflation, pneumothorax, pneumomediastinum, or bleeding.

Brachytherapy

The use of BT has significantly increased as both an adjuvant as well as an alternative radiation option for airway malignancies. There are several advantages of BT over external beam radiation. It can provide a higher dose of radiation to the tumor, minimize the radiation exposure of normal tissue, and dose radiation in a precise location. Because there is a rapid dose "drop-off" with increased distance from the source, there is significantly less injury to the surrounding tissue.

Endobronchial BT is performed by placing the radioactive source through a hollow catheter that is positioned into the endobronchial tree. There is no consensus on the distance prescribed from catheter to tissue, but most authors agree that 1 cm is adequate. The radiation is delivered by an afterloading technique, which involves the placement of a catheter through the bronchoscope to a location that is 2–4 cm distal to the lesion. The catheter is secured, dummy sources are loaded into the catheter, and the radiation dose is calculated. After the position of the catheter is confirmed, the radioactive source replaces the dummy source.

BT can be used by itself or in combination with other endoscopic modalities. Combining laser and BT prolongs symptomatic relief, lessens disease progression, reduces costs, and offers a survival benefit over either modality alone. Aggressive combined therapy with photodynamic therapy (PDT) and BT can improve local tumor control.

The major contraindication of BT is a known fistula to nonbronchial tissue. High-grade obstructions should be debulked prior to BT. It should not be performed in the same endo-bronchial location for six months after the previous full course has been given. The most serious acute complications of BT include fistula formation and massive hemoptysis. Depending on the study reviewed, fistula formation between the airways and other thoracic structures occurred in 1–8 percent of patients. The most feared complication is a fistula formation to the mediastinum. Hemoptysis can occur as either an early complication or late complication. Increased risk factors include increased tumor length, anatomical proximity of the pulmonary artery and major vessels to the lesion (right upper lobe, right main stem bronchus, and left upper lobe), recurrent previously irradiated tumor, increased fraction size, and progression of malignant disease. Other acute complications related to the dose include pneumothorax, bronchospasm, bronchial stenosis, and radiation bronchitis.

Photodynamic Therapy

Endobronchial PDT is emerging as an important treatment for lung cancer. There is sufficient evidence that PDT is safe and effective in treating both early- and late-stage malignancy. In advanced disease, its role is palliative. In early-stage disease, its role is of treatment with curative intent.

PDT involves the administration of an intravenous tumor-specific photosensitizing agent that will either be retained in tumor tissue or have selective toxicity for tumor vasculature. These agents remain inactive until they are activated by laser (monochromatic) light administered by bronchoscopy. After activation, a photochemical reaction occurs that produces reactive oxygen singlets; this reaction results in tumor necrosis. Debridement of the necrotic tissue is then performed bronchoscopically 1–2 days after activation. The most commonly used agent is porfimer sodium, which is a hematoporphyrin derivative.

Contraindications to PDT include allergy to porphyrins and porphyria, tracheal–esophageal fistula, or tumor extension into the esophagus or major blood vessels. Complications of PDT include extreme photosensitivity after the procedure, hemoptysis resulting from tumor necrosis, and possible airway edema postprocedure.

The advantage of PDT is its technical ease and safety. There is minimal risk of perforation and minimal residual effects on the normal tissue. The disadvantages of PDT include the need for "clean-up" bronchoscopies, the need to avoid exposure to sunlight for 4–6 weeks, and the slow onset of action. Because of this, PDT is not appropriate for patients with respiratory distress secondary to obstruction.

Stents

There are a variety of endoscopic interventions available for endoluminal airway obstruction. When obstruction is secondary to extrinsic compression, however, the only sustainable endoscopic procedure available is the placement of a tracheobronchial stent. Stents are essential in maintaining a patent airway in both intrinsic and extrinsic airway obstruction.

Table 16.3 Indications for Tracheobronchial Stents

Malignant Obstruction	Benign Conditions
Extrinsic compression by tumor or lymphadenopathy	Postintubation tracheal stenosis caused by endotracheal or tracheostomy tubes
Endoluminal proliferation of tumors	Anastomotic stenosis after lung transplantation or surgery
Airway maintenance after debulking	Papillomatosis
Closure of tracheobronchial–esophageal fistula with or without esophageal stent	Tracheobronchomalacia
Airway maintenance before radiation and chemotherapy in large occluding tumors affecting central airways	Tracheobronchial stenosis: idiopathic, Wegener's granulomatosis, relapsing polychondritis, tuberculosis, Sjögren's

The main indication for stent placement is relief of symptoms consistent with airway obstruction from either a malignant or benign obstruction that has failed other medical, surgical, or endoscopic therapies. Table 16.3 describes the indications for stent placement.

In malignancy, stents provide excellent sustainable palliation for progressive symptoms in patients whose conditions have been considered terminal. Improved quality of life and functional benefit have been shown in multiple studies. Increased length of survival has been inferred in a few studies. Stent insertion can be an emergent life-saving procedure allowing relief of acute respiratory distress from airway obstruction. It can allow withdrawal from the mechanical ventilator in patients who could not otherwise be extubated.

Over the last 15 years, numerous stents, both metallic and silicone, have evolved from earlier models. Table 16.4 compares characteristics and uses of these two major categories of stents. Metallic stents can be divided into uncovered stainless steel stents (i.e., Gianturco and Palmaz stents) and covered (polyurethane or silicone) stents (i.e., WALLSTENT™, Ultraflex™, and Alveolus™ stents). The covered stents have the benefit of less ingrowth of

Table 16.4 Comparison of Metallic versus Silicone Stents

Metallic Stents	Silicone Stents
Indicated for malignant disease, not indicated in benign disease except as last resource (FDA warning)	Indicated for benign and malignant disease
Inserted with flexible or rigid bronchoscopy	Requires rigid bronchoscopy
Thinner with a greater airway diameter	Thicker with decreased airway diameter
Better able to conform to the airway wall	More difficult to accommodate to an irregular airway narrowing
Fewer secretions problems, especially if the stent is uncovered	Increased secretions
More granulation tissue and mucosal injury	Less mucosal injury and granulation tissue
Difficult and impossible to remove	Easy to remove with rigid bronchoscopy
Difficult to reposition after the stent is in position	Easy to reposition
Migration is common	Migration is common
More expensive	Less expensive
Radiopaque	Not radiopaque
Common brands: Ultraflex® and Alveolus®	Common brands: T tube, Dumon® and Polyflex®

tissue through the mesh of the stent. The silicone stents are available in both straight and Y shapes.

Currently, there is no ideal stent available that would be appropriate for all types of disorders. Excellent results with stents can be achieved in a majority of patients undergoing the procedure if the patient and the particular stent are selected appropriately.

There are many potential complications that can occur when a tracheobronchial stent is placed. Specific complications can be linked to the particular type of stent that is used. Migration is one of the most common complications associated with the use of stents. The silicone stents migrate more easily than the metal stents because, as they are deployed, they return to their preformed shape. When metal stents are deployed, they form more to the wall of the airway.

The proliferation of granulation tissue at the proximal and distal ends of the stent is an obstacle that occurs more frequently with metallic stents, and is thought to be secondary to increased irritation to the mucosa by the metallic wire. An improperly sized stent can lead to a higher incidence of granulation tissue formation because of excessive friction against the wall (too small a stent) or to excessive pressure on the bronchial mucosa (too large a stent). The rate and amount of growth of the tissue vary and can range from very little tissue to total obstruction of the stent, requiring either debridement or even removal of the stent. The location of the stent is thought to be associated with the amount of granulation tissue, with the subglottic area being the worst. Obstruction from this proliferative tissue can occur in only a few weeks. Excessive granulation tissue can decrease mucociliary clearance, which can promote infection.

The silicone stents are known for decreasing mucociliary clearance, which can promote the buildup of secretions. This is not as much of a problem in uncovered metallic stents, because the mesh helps to preserve the clearance. Some suggest that chest physiotherapy and inhaled moisturized air and mucolytic can prevent and/or decrease mucous plugging. Bacterial colonization occurs frequently in patients after stenting; however, this does not necessarily lead to clinical infection.

Stent removal can be complicated with metallic wire stents. Placement of metallic stents should be considered permanent as they are difficult (sometimes impossible) to remove after granulation tissue develops through the wire mesh. If they do need to be removed, they must be removed piece by piece with rigid bronchoscopy. For this reason, silicone stents are usually placed for temporary or benign conditions.

Conclusion

The discipline of interventional pulmonology is advancing quickly as significant developments occur in both the treatment and diagnostic modalities used for airway and pleural disorders. Considerable progress has been made in this field through education, experience, and new discoveries. This chapter focused primarily on the procedures that are currently the most commonly practiced by interventionalists. These techniques make up the foundation of the field. As the field continues to grow, pulmonary interventionalists will be progressively more responsible for a multitude of new procedures that will incorporate palliation, curative treatments, and early diagnosis of these disorders. This will require the collaborative efforts of pulmonologists, thoracic surgeons, radiologists, radiation oncologists, oncologists, and scientists working in both industrial and academic settings. Goals of the procedures, technical details, patient selection criteria, complication prevention and management, and alternative treatment strategies must all be integrated when evaluating and performing these procedures.

Further Readings

Bolliger CT, Mathur P, Beamis JF, et al. ERS/ATS statement on interventional pulmonology. European Respiratory Society/American Thoracic Society. *Eur Respir J.* 2002;19(2):356–373.

Cavaliere S, Venuta F, Foccoli P, Toninelli C, La Face B. Endoscopic treatment of malignant airway obstructions in 2,008 patients [published erratum of serious dosage error appears in *Chest.* 1997; **111**(5):1476]. *Chest.* 1996;110(6):1536–1542.

Chan AL, Yoneda KY, Allen RP, Albertson TE. Advances in the management of endobronchial lung malignancies. *Curr Opin Pulmon Med.* 2003;9(4):301–308.

Coulter TD, Mehta AC. The heat is on: impact of endo-bronchial electrosurgery on the need for Nd-YAG laser photoresection. *Chest.* 2000;118(2):516–521.

Ernst A, Feller-Kopman D, Becker HD, Mehta AC. Central airway obstruction. *Am J Respir Crit Care Med.* 2004;169(12):1278–1297.

Hautmann H, Gamarra F, Pfeifer KJ, Huber RM. Fiberoptic bronchoscopic balloon dilatation in malignant tracheobronchial disease: indications and results. *Chest.* 2001;120(1):43–49.

Homasson JP. Bronchoscopic cryotherapy. *J Bronchol.* 1995;2:145–149.

Lee P, Kupeli E, Mehta AC. Therapeutic bronchoscopy in lung cancer. Laser therapy, electrocautery, brachytherapy, stents, and photodynamic therapy. *Clin Chest Med.* 2002;23(1):241–256.

Mehrishi S, Ost D. Photodynamic therapy. *J Bronchol.* 2002;9(3):218–222.

Rafanan AL, Mehta AC. Stenting of the tracheobronchial tree. *Radiol Clin North Am.* 2000;38(2):395–408.

Saad CP, Murthy S, Krizmanich G, Mehta AC. Self-expandable metallic airway stents and flexible bronchoscopy: long-term outcomes analysis. *Chest.* 2003;124(5):1993–1999.

Seijo LM, Sterman DH. Interventional pulmonology. *N Engl J Med.* 2001;344(10):740–792.

Turner JF Jr, Wang KP. Endobronchial laser therapy. *Clin Chest Med.* 1999;20(1):107–122.

Index